THE
POWER
OF THE
VOICE

THE POWER OF THE VOICE

Jean Abitbol, MD

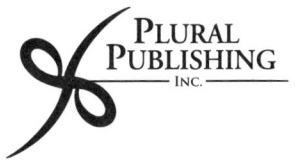

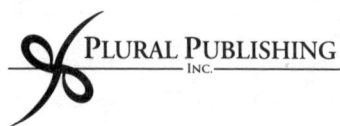

5521 Ruffin Road
San Diego, CA 92123

email: info@pluralpublishing.com
website: http://www.pluralpublishing.com

Le Pouvoir de la Voix © 2016 Allary Éditions
Published by special arrangement with Allary Éditions in conjunction with their duly appointed agent 2 Seas Literary Agency.

Typeset in 11/14 Palatino by Flanagan's Publishing Services, Inc.
Printed in the United States of America by McNaughton & Gunn, Inc.

All rights, including that of translation, reserved. No part of this publication may be reproduced, stored in a retrieval system, or transmitted in any form or by any means, electronic, mechanical, recording, or otherwise, including photocopying, recording, taping, Web distribution, or information storage and retrieval systems without the prior written consent of the publisher.

For permission to use material from this text, contact us by
Telephone: (866) 758-7251
Fax: (888) 758-7255
E-mail: permissions@pluralpublishing.com

Every attempt has been made to contact the copyright holders for material originally printed in another source. If any have been inadvertently overlooked, the publishers will gladly make the necessary arrangements at the first opportunity.

Library of Congress Cataloging-in-Publication Data

Names: Abitbol, Jean, author.
Title: The power of the voice / Jean Abitbol.
Other titles: Pouvoir de la voix. English
Description: San Diego, CA : Plural, 2017. | Includes bibliographical references and index.
Identifiers: LCCN 2017030952 | ISBN 9781635500547 (alk. paper) | ISBN 1635500540 (alk. paper)
Subjects: | MESH: Voice | Speech | Verbal Behavior
Classification: LCC QP306 | NLM WV 501 | DDC 612.78—dc23
LC record available at https://lccn.loc.gov/2017030952

CONTENTS

Foreword   *vii*
Introduction   *xi*
Acknowledgments   *xv*

1 The Voice as an Instrument   1

2 The Voices of Power   55

3 The Essential Is Invisible   99

4 The Voice Must Go On   111

5 The Voices of Silence   147

Conclusion   *165*

FOREWORD

It all began one Christmas Eve, in 1978. Back then, I was in my first year of residency. I was a resident in surgery at a general hospital near Paris and, as luck would have it, for my first December 24 night as a surgeon in the hospital. That night, I was on duty in the emergency room. No time for a Christmas truce! Indeed, due to the usual high number of accidents on Christmas Eve, it was one of the busiest shifts of the year. It didn't help that back then, wearing a seat belt wasn't yet compulsory. Around 6 a.m., a 23-year-old female was admitted in the emergency room and directly transferred to the intensive care unit. She had multiple contusions and respiratory distress. Her abdomen was supple, there was no internal bleeding, but both jaw and larynx appeared to be fractured, as confirmed later by X-ray. She was barely conscious. Of course, restoring her breathing capacity was a priority, but I found myself unexpectedly just as concerned about ensuring the young woman didn't lose her ability to speak!

Now here we are:

Her blood oxygen level was sinking fast. To restore it to normal levels, we needed to urgently transfer her to the operating room to intubate her. In the operating room on the first floor, the surgical lights were already on. The young woman's blood oxygen levels were down to 87%. The fractures of the larynx and the mandible ruled out intubation. Our only option was a tracheotomy: a lifesaving incision under the Adam's apple. The chief operating room nurse assisting me told me what I already knew: "Mr. Abitbol, we have to perform a tracheotomy urgently, I'll help you and we can't wait for your colleagues." The anesthetist backed her on this. We got started. But they did not know that I had never done a tracheotomy! To be on the safe side, I asked them to beep the chief resident: He was busy operating on a fractured femur. I then called the assistant resident: He was operating on a ruptured spleen. In despair, I asked that the associate professor of ENT be advised: He was also operating. I knew how to perform this life-saving procedure, which I was taught in Paris on the sixth floor of the medical school in Rue des Saint-Pères on cadavers and practised on cadavers at the morgue at the medical institute near the Quai de la Rapée located along the River Seine embankment. So, this was my first "live" tracheotomy. By now my patient was close to heart failure. I had to take action. Minutes later, having donned scrubs and surgical gloves, I was disinfecting the surgical field. I palpated the neck, searching for the thyroid cartilage, and two fingers higher, I felt the cricothyroid membrane and the cricoid, the ring of cartilage that surrounds the trachea. I pressed down on the membrane with my index and, holding my breath, made an incision just above it, at the tip of my index finger. All was well, the trachea was now open, and I could intubate. Moments later, the associate professor joined me and together we completed the intervention, applying ourselves to rebuilding the jaw and the larynx. My initial concern hadn't abated and I shared it with the professor. "Do you think this young woman will be able to speak again?" "For sure, no reason why not," he answers. I then asked him which department might best help me perfect my technique and master the tracheotomy. "Why young man, the ENT department of course!" And that is how I discovered my vocation, on a Christmas Eve shift in 1978. I decided then and there to devote myself to the science and art of the voice and ear.

After the operation, I sought out the woman's fiancé to reassure him and discover how the accident came about. Heading for home after Christmas Eve celebrations with the family, he lost control of his Peugeot 204 on an icy patch of road and slammed straight into a tree at 60 mph. I saw the couple again three months later. The young woman had recovered her voice, and a beautiful one at that.

After 18 months of general surgery internship in Amiens, I decided to become an ENT specialist. At the end of 1978, I joined the staff of the Hôpital Foch, in Paris. I'm lucky: Laser technology had just made its appearance, and Foch was the first hospital in Europe to adopt this revolutionary invention. Gaining hands-on experience as a young surgeon, the laser accompanied my every step, allowing me to discover both the world of microsurgery and the world of laryngology, a specialty dealing with science and emotion: the voice.

In June 1980, I visited for the first time The Voice Foundation in New York, where I had a lucky break. I met the master: Doctor Wilbur James Gould and his chief resident Robert Thayer Sataloff, who has since been my best friend for almost 40 years. In the context of the Juilliard School, a performing arts conservatory of international fame and a holy temple of research into the human voice, Gould had hatched the brilliant idea of bringing together physicists, ENT specialists, surgeons, acousticians, and voice performers under one roof for a seven-day conference. He had understood the potential of such a diversity of talents, and by opening up the various disciplines that focused on different aspects of the voice, he succeeded in creating a meeting of minds that transcended them. The lesson I took away from this served me throughout my life and career. Since then, I have never missed the opportunity to attend in June this remarkable brainstorming event at which art and science fuse so seamlessly.

In 1984, I produced *L'Empreinte vocal* (*The Vocal Imprint*) a 16-mm documentary film lasting 27 minutes. In it, I presented the technology for exploring the larynx and the voice, using voice performers such as the Golden Gate Quartet; Clyde Wright was the tenor or the Gipsy Kings in their early days. I put the film in a red box, intending to show it to Professor Gould.

To be honest, I found this a daunting prospect, but Gould's response was disconcertingly straightforward. Not only did he agree to view my film, but he also suggested that three of his co-chairmen attend the viewing: G. Paul Moore, Friedrich Brodnitz, and Hans von Leden, who were the kings of voice science in the United States, the original roots team of The Voice Foundation. Without further ado, the viewing was set for the following Tuesday, in the auditorium, between 12 and 2 p.m., during the lunch break.

I have to admit the enthusiastic reaction of these distinguished researchers took me by surprise. Gould immediately invited me to show the documentary in a plenary session, a true consecration of my work, more precious to me than any prize could be. *The Vocal Imprint* was subsequently voted best documentary at the international festival of medical films in Paris in 1985. The prize was awarded by then Minister of Health, Georgina Dufoix, and was shown in more than 17 countries. It is still available at the Voice Foundation.

I started out my medical career as a surgeon, then practiced as an otolaryngologist specializing in head and neck surgery while gaining experience in phoniatrics, the medical specialty dealing with voice problems. My exposure to the Voice Foundation was without a doubt the trigger that set me on the path to becoming the specialist I am today as not only an ENT but, as we say in France, a phoniatrician since 1990. My predilection for a multidisciplinary approach was born there, and it made me realize that the doctor dealing with voice has to be a fan of voice professionals, because voice surgery deals first and foremost with emotions.

As I navigated the worlds of science, medicine, and vocal emotion, my path was studded with scientific adventures, singular meetings, and remarkable stories. Initially, I set out to understand the origins of the human voice. That gave rise to my first book, *The Odyssey of the Voice* (Plural Publishing, 2006; translated from *L'Odyssée de la Voix*, second Edition Flammarion, «Champs Sciences», 2013).

In it, I invite the reader on a wonderful journey getting to know the evolution of our planet and of our DNA with the Foxp2 gene of the voice, the origins of the voice in *Homo sapiens* and the differences between man and other primates that have enabled humans to speak. But the same passion I nursed for the human voice led me to want to get to the bottom of another question that was haunting me: How does the voice hold so much sway? How come the voice has such a power? Is it the power of the voice that gives the power to our leaders?

INTRODUCTION

Our Voice Empowers Us!

Man possesses a rare treasure: the human voice. It connects all human beings on Planet Earth. It underpins our past, as it wills our future. We're all children of the human voice. Throughout the centuries, it has ensured the survival of our species, fascinating scientists, philosophers, intellectuals, and artists.

The voice isn't just a communication tool; it also allows us to be creative, and it shapes our thoughts and gives expression to our emotions. From the dawn of history to the modern day, the voice has always captivated the minds of men.

Our voice can make our fortune or spell disaster for us. The result of an alchemy of mind and body, it is an instrument for persuasion, seduction, and charm, and it reflects our personality and our true self. In *The Sacred Night*, Tahar Ben Jelloun writes, "You can't lie to a blind person; you can spin a yarn, but the blind will lend more credence to your voice than to the words spoken."

Between chaos and harmony, coalescing the real and the virtual, body and soul, the human voice is singular, yet universal. Like a fingerprint, common to mankind, yet unique to each of us.

An integral part of our life and of our past, the voice is a common marker of our history, an essential link between our emotions, our imagination, and our reason. It allows us to both interact with our environment and to evolve within it.

Though our voice reflects our true self, it is also our secret garden. Indeed, it allows us to build relationships but also animates an internal dialogue that is hermetic to others. In that inner silence, our voice is never quiet; it never forsakes us, constantly prodding us, capable of instilling in us the life force that moves us on, guiding our actions and forging our intuition. *Voice is both immanence and transcendence.*

Today, the voice metamorphoses into writing. We talk to a computer and it transcribes the sounds into written form. The power of the voice is impressive, its sway far beyond what was thought possible half a century ago. Where there is voice, there is life. Once enunciated, things spring into existence. Our voice is a writing instrument for our thoughts, a virtual hyphen between the conscious and the unconscious mind. Both flagship and pilot boat of our imagination, its power is amazing, leading us at times, much to our surprise, into new territories and in roads of our mind that at the beginning of our talk we did not expect at all.

The voice can be used offensively or defensively. It is a weapon of seduction or of mass destruction. It is the archer, the bow, and the arrow rolled into one. The voice is Satan when the archer is Hitler, Venus when the archer is Cupid.

An intrinsic part of our daily life, it is so omnipresent that we take it for granted and treat it with indifference, until the day it fails us, and then we miss it. It just is! Stress or straining the voice can impair it, as can diseases, and the resulting voice disorders and dysphonia bring in a break with the outside world. When our voice is broken or hoarse, croaky or raspy, injured or faint, it loses all its power, dispossessed of its influence over its owner and over others. When the voice returns after such an eclipse, it brings light back into our life and we cherish it like a human being, like someone we care for, with wonderment and relief, glad that this imposed, wretched silence is over. Indeed, we refer to our voice as if it were another person: "I've lost my voice," "I don't know what's happened to my voice," and "I never thought that my voice can leave me like this."

Since time immemorial, human beings have forged primary emotional ties with each other thanks to the voice. It affects every aspect of our existence. It is a cornerstone of any society, enabling us to network, to connect with the outside world, and to integrate ourselves in it. The voice is a mainstay for man's self, soul, and very existence.

From the ancient agora to the television screen, the voice wields its influence over all human matters, be they of a legal, political, commercial, artistic, or romantic nature.

When we read a book, we're at liberty to stop at any point, to return to an earlier section or to make annotations. The voice doesn't allow us that freedom. We're swept along by the unfolding narration, by the avalanche of words, by the musicality of the sentence; we're hooked because they soothe us, move us, or stimulate us. Such is the power of the voice, a power that isn't without danger, because a voice can captivate its listeners and transport them into the speaker's affective universe, impeding their capacity to reason and making them susceptible to archaic reflexes that appeal to their reptilian, primitive brain.

The voice, source of our life force and power, can bring for us and in us sunshine, shadows, twilight, or dawn. It regulates the rhythm of our silences. It reflects our state of mind, the scars left by our experiences, our individual space-time continuum. The voice is the past, the present, and the future at the same time.

As a doctor and surgeon with a deep passion for the human voice, let me take you in the ship of the intricacies of the human voice between thunder and calm, not just in its scientific and medical dimensions, but also in its political dimensions, from mentor to tyrant, in its spiritual and artistic dimensions, from preacher to singer, and, in its esthetic dimensions, from sensuality to seduction. I propose to take you on a journey that will reveal to you the alchemy that occurs between our emotions and our reason at the heart of our imperceptible and irrational vibrations. I will take you deep into the kingdom of the voice, of which the larynx is the Holy Grail; and unveiling for you the secret of its power.

ACKNOWLEDGMENTS

What a pleasure it has been writing this book, not only because this was an outlet for my passion for the human voice but also because of the many people I met thanks to them and, above all, the voice professionals, with whom I had numerous discussions about the power of the voice, discussions that were often very emotional.

Thankful

To my children, Delphine and Patrick, always present when needed for commenting; their objectivity, goodwill, love, and affection.

To Yves Gauguet, a philosopher, for his loyal friendship throughout the penning of this book. Always available, he gave me generous advice and encouragement.

To Doctor Jean-Jacques Maimaran, who has been by my side for over 30 years.

To Cynthia, my efficient and dedicated assistant, who was able to adapt herself to my medical and literary universe.

To Nathalie, whose presence, support, pertinent remarks, and valuable insights meant so much to me.

To the scientific friends of the American Voice Foundation, with a warm special thanks to Robert Sataloff, Mike Benninger, and Thomas Murry.

My gratitude goes to the following people, be they philosophers or men of law, singers or actors, scientists or entertainers:

To Jean-Luc Kandyoti, accomplished pianist and composer; thanks to whom I was able to better address the correspondence between the voice, our very own musical instrument, and the musical work by Beethoven or Bach and Jazz.

To Mr. Robert Badinter, former President of the Constitutional Council, and former Minister of Justice, who helped me to better detect, understand, and analyze the complex and sometimes conflicting relationship between individual and collective feeling.

To Pierre Cycman, lawyer, and to Thierry Tordjman, lawyer, my nephew, who many times gave me valuable insights into the strong relationship between science and the power of the voice. Peter Brook, a true director of voices, and Robert Hossein and Gérard Darmon, whose voices are the star, and Charles Aznavour, who challenges the march of time.

To Garou, whose voice challenges the laws of science by forcing his voice without ever damaging it. Angélique Kidjo, whose voices are universal and so unique. Ruggero Raimondi, Florent Pagny, Mika, and Hélène Ségara, whose voices resonate in tune to the inner vibrations of their auditors.

To the impersonators, voice illusionists, artists of artists: Michaël Gergorio, Véronic Dicaire, and Liane Foly; Laurent Gerra, unintentional scientist, whose vocal spectrograph is acoustically so amazingly close to that of the politicians he imitates.

To the ventriloquists, magicians of the voice, represented so remarkably by Jeff Dunham, Jeff Panacloc, and Marc Métral. A special thanks to Christian Gabriel: He has helped my research for years.

To André Dussollier, actor, and, unbeknown to him, a scientist exploring the future of the voice.

To Céline Dion, whose voice is to variety what the voice of Maria Callas is to opera.

To Malcy Ozannat and Nicole Lattès, who have provided encouragement for this book and for their thoughtfulness, who understand the hidden meaning of words and for their forbearance.

To voice performers

CHAPTER 1

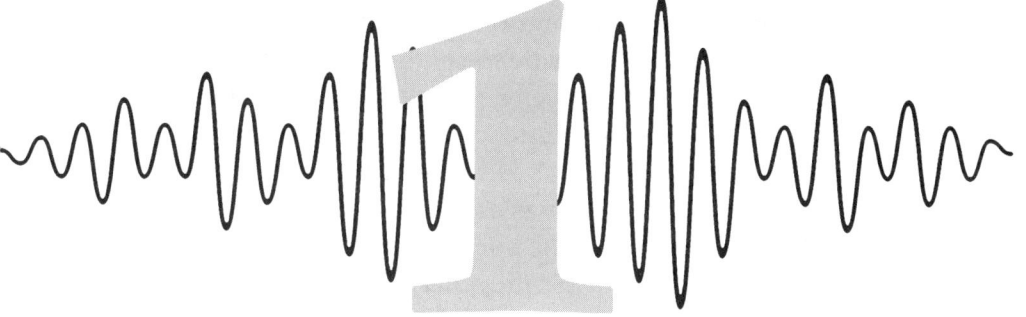

The Voice as an Instrument

The Voice Under Observation

For over 10,000 years, the voice was considered to be the ether of life by all civilizations, from the Dogon to the Aborigines, from the Egyptians to the Greeks, from the Arab civilization to the Age of Enlightenment. It was only in the 19th century that the voice was revealed as an entity that could be analyzed scientifically.

Manuel García's Cane or the Grail of the Voice

On a beautiful autumn day in 1854, Manuel García took a sunlit stroll through the gardens of the Palais-Royal, in Paris. Approaching 50, this dapper man was an eminent professor of singing at the

Royal Academy of Music in London. Engrossed by the glinting reflections of the sun on the silver pommel of his cane, he seemed quite oblivious of the nearby residence of the Duke of Orléans or the crowded cafés patronized by the elite of his day.

Manuel García was no doctor, yet his knowledge of anatomy was impressive. He had on occasion dissected larynxes at a medical school, but the larynx of a dead person doesn't vibrate and it reveals nothing of the workings of the spoken or singing voice. Staring at the reflections on the pommel of his cane, he suddenly had a brainwave: Why not use the reflections of the sun on a mirror to examine a person's throat? Without further ado, he set off for the premises of *"Etablissements Charrière,"* makers of surgical instruments near the Saint Germain des Pres and Saint Michel at the Odéon. He purchased a dental mirror costing six francs. Back home, he devised a system for observing the vocal cords and immediately tried it out on himself.

He practiced scales, from the highest to the lowest registers, laughed and coughed, all the while noting the mobility of his vocal cords: They separated when he breathed and came together when he spoke, coughed, or faked crying. This is the mechanism that enables sounds to be produced deep in the throat. As Manuel García observed the voice in action up close, he felt as if he had discovered the Holy Grail of the human voice. A new science and branch of medicine was born: laryngology!

Manuel García died in 1905, aged 101. He left behind a groundbreaking tome: *A Complete Treatise on the Art of Singing*. In this historic book, published in 1847, he laid down the first rules of phonation, thus continuing the García family tradition of outstanding accomplishments in the sphere of the voice.

Manuel Garcia had two sisters: María Malibran, an exceptional opera diva in her day, and Pauline Viardot, an eminent singing teacher.

The laryngeal mirror invented by Manuel García over a century and a half ago remains to this day one of the key tools used by laryngologists. To him we owe being able to observe someone's vocal cords by pressing down on a person's tongue while he or she says "Ahh . . . ."

The Cathedral of the Voice

When "observing the voice," one has the impression of entering a vocal cathedral. The science of phoniatry experienced its second quantum leap in 1981, first with the advent of the revolutionary videostroboscope. This objective and replicable observation technique analyzes chronologically the kinetic variations of the larynx and thus enabling a precise decryption of vocal pathologies during singing and talking. That same year, I perfected a technique of vocal dynamic exploration that conjugated several aspects of laryngeal observation: pharyngolaryngeal video endoscopy. One could at long last observe the voice speaking and singing. Introduced via the nose, the endoscope reveals the mobility of the vocal tract, without any of the interference that results from introducing an instrument via the mouth coupled with the electrolaryngograph done by Adrian Fourcin. Back then, the frame rate when filming the voice was 25 images per second. In 2000, pharyngolaryngeal video endoscopies achieved a frame rate of 4,000 images per second. The scientific fallout from this has been outstanding. This dynamic exploration of the voice establishes the identity card of the voice: its "voiceprint."

The tone of a voice, also known as its color, is highly individual and difficult to define. It is one of the principal characteristics of the voiceprint. Likewise in music: The same note played on a violin and on a saxophone will sound quite different, even when played in the same frequency. Indeed, each instrument has its own signature, even within a family of instruments: the acoustics of a Stradivarius, composed of 71 pieces of wood stringently selected for their specificity, will be very different from those of a simple violin for budding musicians, because it is the body of the violin, its resonance chamber, that enhances the radiated tonality. The human voice is subject to the same kind of effect. The timbre that characterizes a person's voice is shaped by the passage of the voice through the different resonance chambers situated above the vocal cords.

The most impressive feature of this vocal resonance is its harmonic content. Harmonics amplify the voice and embellish its quality: They're natural "amplifiers" and "embellishers" of the human voice, acting as an "equalizer" for the instrument of the voice, which is both a string instrument and a wind instrument. Vocal sounds have been measured since 1936, thanks to the development of spectrographic analysis in France by Jean Tarnaud.

We're not created equal regarding our vocal capabilities. Some of the greatest vocalists, such as Luciano Pavarotti, can produce seven harmonics, whereas the average man can only produce three! How is it that a Maria Callas, a Mario Del Monaco, or a Caruso is able to deliver so much emotional vibration? It is because when they emit a fundamental frequency ($f0$ or $f\ zero$) by vibrating their vocal cords, they immediately create secondary fundamental tones, known as harmonics. Certain harmonics are more powerful than others thanks to their reverberation in the resonance chambers. These stronger harmonics are known as formants.

Origins of the Voice, of Language, and of the Mother Tongue

Frederick the Second and the Wild Children

The articulated voice isn't innate. Even though from birth, we're able to babble forth sounds, vowels, and consonants, these don't have meaning, nor do they form a language. Or, do they? Does a primitive mother language exist before language, as we know it? In the 13th century, Frederick II of Hohenstaufen was the Holy Roman Emperor of Sicily, Germany, and Jerusalem from 1220 to 1250. He did speak six languages: Latin, Sicilian, German, French, Greek, and Arabic. He was also learning Hebrew. He carried out an experiment to trace the origin of language. The Polish author Gustaw Herling-Grudzinski refers to it as, "Seven outlandish episodes marked the reign of the emperor Frederick II. The second outlandish episode occurred when he decided to find out what language children would speak if from birth, and for some years, they heard no words spoken."

Unscrupulous and thirsty for knowledge, this legendary emperor, erudite and on occasion cruel, concocted an experiment to pierce the mystery of the human voice. He ordered several newborn babies to be brought to his palace. There they were isolated from each other, and their nannies and suckling nurses were instructed to breastfeed them, care for them, and bathe them, without ever addressing a word to them. Under such conditions, deprived of a mother tongue and with no social interaction, what language would these children speak: Hebrew, Aramaic (believed by the emperor to be the original language of humanity), Greek, Latin, Arabic, German, or simply the language of their parents?

After four years of this isolation, the children were returned to a normal life, with social interaction. They seemed to behave normally, but not one of them spoke! They just mumbled incoherently. Yet they had all the characteristics of *Homo sapiens* with the mechanical structure for speaking in place, a developed brain, they stood upright, and could walk. But they had no voice. The voice remained an unchartered territory for these wild children, who never learned the basics of any language! Deprived of language, *Homo sapiens* are no better and no worse than a chimpanzee in a three-piece suit. But the case of these children is worse than first appears. It became chillingly obvious that the potential for even primitive communication was lacking and they all died before reaching adulthood. Does the voice, then, condition our very survival? Herling concludes, "The truth is that children can't survive if their carers don't talk to them, smile at them and cuddle them. A human life is built on words and by the Word and conditioned by words and for the Word." Man's progeny is a social animal, its brain is nourished by the human voice, and social interaction is critical to its survival.

For millions of years, the chances of survival of human beings have indubitably been influenced by their intraspecies communication and exchanges, the foundation of which is the human voice.

Alice and Shiguru

Having disproved the possible existence of an original primitive tongue, the notion of the mother tongue remains to be explored.

The case of Alice and Shiguru springs to mind. Aged nine and 11, respectively, their parents bring them to me for a banal pharyngitis consultation. The father is Japanese but speaks French fluently with barely a trace of an accent. The mother is French. After spending nearly five years in Japan, the family has been back in France for two years. The children have therefore been raised in a bilingual culture. Their throat problem is soon forgotten as they bombard me, in perfect French, with questions about my settings: computers, cameras, spectrographs, and endo-videoscopes. Faced with these keen, smart youngsters, I'm happy to satisfy their curiosity. Intrigued by their linguistic assimilation, I ask them which language they feel more comfortable in. It turns out they're just as happy speaking Japanese as French. "But what language do you speak to each other in?" Alice answers, "French mostly, but if we don't want others to understand what we're saying, at school or when we're at a friend's home, then we switch to Japanese." Shigeru agrees and then adds, "When we quarrel, I speak Japanese." He finds Japanese a more forceful, expressive, and more empowering language and speaks it when he needs to assert or defend himself.

I ask them to pass a fairly simple test—quick mental calculations—to help determine whether they have a mother tongue plus a secondary tongue or two mother tongues. People are consistently faster doing mental computations in their mother tongue than in a secondary tongue. Yet these siblings are equally fast in both Japanese and French; they answer on the button, with the same delay. They definitely have two mother tongues. When I retest them in English, which they also speak, I observe a slight latency of a few seconds: they're translating the numbers mentally into one of their two mother tongues before answering.

The human voice and the mother tongue etch themselves onto the cerebral cortex of a child, like an indelible tattoo, from the age of 18 months until the fourth year. If, from infancy, a child learns two languages in parallel, the two areas of the brain monitoring those languages will also develop in parallel. In 1997, K. H. S. Kim, et al, of Cornell University, published in *Nature* that the brain of someone brought up bilingually since birth involves Wernicke's area and Broca's area and are practically superimposed. However, if a second language is learned after the age of four, it doesn't manifest in the same area of the brain. It was demonstrated with positron emission tomography (PET scan) and functional nuclear magnetic resonance imaging (MRI), during vocalization exercises.

It is tempting to assume there is an analogy between bilingual children and ambidextrous children, but there isn't. A study carried out by T. J. Crow et al. in 2007 with 11,600 children over the age of 11 showed that right-handed children who are left-brain dominant learn languages faster than ambidextrous children who are left-brain dominant. The power of the voice is therefore also influenced by our laterality.

When functional MRI is used to examine the brain of ambidextrous subjects, it reveals defective laterality in the areas that monitor language. The left and right hemispheres are practically symmetrical, with the language function duplicated. There seems to be a "true" area of Broca in the left hemisphere and a "pseudo" area of Broca's area in the right hemisphere. This is anarchy, or something approaching anarchy: There are two orchestra conductors! This genetic predisposition can have serious consequences. Could it present the risk of vocal schizophrenia? Schizophrenia happens to be 20 times more frequent in the ambidextrous population than in the non-ambidextrous population. In the latter, as a rule, one hemisphere is hypertrophied. One of the genes that ensures this beneficial asymmetry is located at the level of sex chromosome X. Turner syndrome, a genetic anomaly in which each cell has only one copy of the X chromosome instead of the usual two—resulting in XO instead of XX—is associated with a high incidence of schizophrenia and practically no evidence of cerebral asymmetry. Moreover, the perception of language is disturbed. It seems therefore that cerebral asymmetry is a capital element underpinning the potential of the voice in *Homo sapiens*. Dorothy Bishop did a superb study on cerebral asymmetry and language development. In most people, language is processed predominantly by the left hemisphere, but we don't know how or why. A popular view is that developmental language disorders result from a poorly lateralized brain, but until recently, evidence has been weak and indirect. Modern neuroimaging methods have made it possible to study normal and abnormal development of lateralized function in the developing brain and have confirmed links with language and literacy impairments.

Mario

Bilingual children must imperatively continue to use both their mother tongues if they're to maintain their multilingualism. Mental stimulation is the bedrock of knowledge, of memory, of evolution. If one stops using a language, the neuronal circuitry for that language fades out, as Mario's extraordinary case reveals.

Mario had consulted me for a persistent hoarse throat that bothered him. Aged 75, the man is a deep bass opera singer and a theater actor. There was a polyp on his right vocal cord. Using laryngeal endoscopy, I performed laser microsurgery on him under general anesthetic. The operation went well, there was no bleeding whatsoever, and the postoperative result was satisfactory. The polyp proved to be benign. Mario was transferred to the recovery room. I passed by to see him before taking him back to his room and asked him, "How do you feel?" Mario answered me in a language I couldn't understand. What happened? I asked myself. My concern was, did the operation induce a stroke? I asked the nurse to summon a neurologist. As far as I can tell, Mario was delirious. But to my surprise, the nurse could understand him. "Dr Abitbol, he hasn't had a stroke, he's just speaking Greek!" "But he isn't Greek, as far as I know, I've known him for years!" At the end of my surgical morning, I returned to his room. Mario was speaking French again. He questioned me about his polyp. "Have I got cancer?" I reassured him, "It's just a benign lesion." I did not want to go further on the "Greek" mystery.

A week later, during his postoperative follow-up, I asked Mario if he was of Greek origin. He hesitated, pondering my question, before answering, "No, I am not Greek! But why do you ask me? A few seconds later he said, "As a matter of fact, I was born in Salonika. My father was Greek, but I hardly knew him. He died when I was five and my mother, who was French, returned to live in Paris. This was nearly 70 years ago!" I told him about the incident in the recovery room. "But I hardly know my mother tongue!" he exclaimed.

Most likely, the general anesthetic induced a very slight decrease in oxygen levels precisely in the area of the brain that monitors language. Being more vascularized, the older "Greek" layer—the mother tongue—recovered its normal oxygenation levels first. Thus, this part of the brain had kept its integrity, its memory bank, and its linguistic dictionary intact for nearly 70 years. I asked him when he last spoke Greek and he replied, "Doctor, I left Greece over 70 years ago. I grew up in France in an artistic background, speaking only French, though I have on occasion sung in Greek."

A one-year-old bilingual infant can discern the musicality specific to a language and registers it permanently in their brain. This isn't due to a special gift or to any genetic predisposition the left or right brain may have; rather, it is proof that right from infancy, the brain is able to assimilate the human voice, music, and verbal utterances. The only thing the brain needs, straight from birth, is auditory stimulation and, later, stimulation from the audiophonatory loop.

The brain of a newborn contains the seeds of all possible phonemes, a complete polychromatic spectrum of all languages, but in most cases, if they aren't used or activated, the child loses them after the age of seven. If children learn a foreign language after the age of five, invariably they unconsciously superimpose on it the rhythm of their mother tongue and they speak it with a "foreign" accent.

The Maternal Voice

A baby is under the influence of its mother's voice long before its birth. The fetus hears the heartbeats of its mother, a three-stroke beat that is music to its ears, conveying security and protection.

Six months after its birth, a typical developing baby is able to recognize the vowels of its mother tongue and, more specifically, the musicality of these vowels and the intonation of its mother tongue. By nine months old, it can form words by linking two phonemes; at 18 months, it can organize words; as a two-year-old toddler, it can build sentences; and and at three, it already has a grasp of basic grammar.

We know that the voice contributes to social interaction in many vertebrates, but less is known about the hormonal mechanisms that are triggered when an infant hears its mother's voice. What role do these hormones play in our behavioral evolution? Oxytocin is a singular hormone that plays a significant role in several social behaviors, notably in mother-child bonding and in the suppression of stress in the presence of relatives, hence its reputation as "the love hormone." Cortisol is another hormone secreted by our body that increases during stress conditions.

Leslie Seltzer, a biological anthropologist from the University of Wisconsin-Madison, was keen to evaluate the influence of the mother's voice on her child during a stressful episode. Children recognize the mother's voice with her own specific words, the right rhythm, and the music of her unique vibrations when life seems to be getting too much. Now it seems her voice on the phone can work the same soothing magic as when she is there in person to give her offspring comfort. Seltzer did a study on 61 girls aged seven to 12. The children had to make an impromptu speech and solve mathematical problems in front of strangers.

This protocol increased both the heart rate and levels of cortisol of the girls. But what about the oxytocin?

The girls were split into three groups:

1. Girls in the first group could see their mother straight after their performance, and she reassured them both verbally and physically.
2. Girls in the second group were handed a cell phone and mom was on the line to speak with them.
3. Girls in the third group didn't see their mother or listen to her; instead, they watched a 75-minute film deemed to be emotionally neutral, the *March of the Penguins*.

Oxytocin increased intensively with a similar level in the first and second groups. By the time the children of these two groups went home, they were still enjoying the benefits of this relief and their cortisol levels still low. A simple telephone call could have turned on this physiological effect. The contact with the mother's voice made these girls produce oxytocin, which brought their stress level down. In the third group, the girls had no contact with their mother and were still stressed out. They showed no oxytocin production and a considerable increase in cortisol.

The test was done using saliva and urine. But, as we could have guessed, as the oxytocin presence grew, cortisol faded. In her report, Seltzer, who led the research, said, "The children who got to interact with their mothers had virtually the same hormonal response, whether they interacted in person or over the phone. It was understood that oxytocin release in the context of social bonding usually required physical contact. But it's clear from these results that a mother's voice can have the same effect as a hug, even if they're not standing there." Isn't it the power of the mother's voice?

Why weren't any boys used in the study? Oxytocin responses are stronger in females than in males. In adult women, the hormone plays a role in labor, preparing for birth, and breastfeeding.

Seltzer's results show that in social interactions, both the human voice and physical contact have equal influence on hormonal regulation. This could provide early clues as to the biological basis for the success of cell phones. The love hormone, on cue with a simple phone call!

Evidence indeed. Children retain the memory of the tone and vibrations of their mother's voice from the womb. Hence, when that voice changes, the family dynamics can be seriously thrown.

I recall the case of Mrs. H, a 37-year-old woman who consulted me. She spoke with a thin, faint voice, without forcing. I asked her to cough and her cough made no sound. This is an unmistakable symptom, since a cough is normally audible because the two vocal cords touch each other and in effect "smack" together.

My patient specified that she lost her voice suddenly at the age of 13, after coming down with the flu, and that it was never the same again. She was now used to her altered voice but wished to recover her normal voice. "I have two children, aged seven and nine. Their bedroom is on the first floor. To call them, I must ring a little hand bell or else press a service bell in the kitchen. And, talking on the phone is just beyond me now." When I observed her larynx, I found that the right vocal cord was mobile and moved perfectly to join the medial part of the glottal space. But the left vocal cord was paralyzed, stuck far off from the center of the glottis space of the larynx. In our jargon, we call this "abductor paralysis." Since the vocal cords can't have contact, the vibration of both vocal cords is impossible, like a bow on the string of the violin. If the bow doesn't touch the string, there is no sound. Here the voice was barely audible and Mrs. H. was reduced to whispering. I suggested a procedure that would enable the two cords to come together during phonation. It is a simple matter of medializing the left vocal cord, positioning it in such a way that the right vocal cord can meet the opposite one and thereby produce the vibration that is the source of vocal sound. We achieve this by injecting the left vocal cord with a product that creates an augmentation. Now they have contact to produce a sound. The procedure is done under general anesthetic; a laryngoscope is introduced orally and microsurgery is performed. Five to 10 days later, the voice is back to normal. Mrs. H. thought it over, and then agreed to the intervention. I operated on the larynx of Mrs. H. a week later. She has recovered a beautiful voice, feminine and tonic. She let me in on an incredible admission: "I never got to know my grown-up voice, my real voice, a feminine voice!" But two weeks later, Mrs. H. was back with her husband and two children. They all looked at me as if I did something wrong. The older child complained, "I can't recognize my mother anymore, what did you do to her?" "This isn't the woman I married, I don't recognize her either," Mr. H. concurred. As far as her relatives were concerned, her feeble vocal tonality was her normal voice, and it looked like I had metamorphosed her. I had to exert considerable educational skills to reassure and convince them they would get used to her voice. Still, the family's dismay is perfectly understandable, especially the children's distress. They had to deal with both the loss of their mother's former voice and the switch to a substitute "new" voice that, in fact, was their mother's almost authentic voice, which just goes to show that "a normal voice" does not mean much but it is still a mark.

Mirror Neurons

One thing is certain, when learning to speak, our mental resources aren't focalized on a highly rational and objective one-way process. We are engaging in a spontaneous and sincere exchange with another being, in which our memory is stirred by our emotions. It requires us being in tune with other people's intentions and internalizing their movements and thought processes. We may imagine the important role of mirror neurons about the human voice and its power.

The discovery of "mirror neurons" by neurologists Vittorio Gallese and Giacomo Rizzolatti brought about a better understanding of the mechanism inherent in social cognition, in all that pertains to learning by imitation, to affective processes, to understanding others, to emotion and empathy.

These mirror neurons can be observed in action when one subject either observes a second subject perform a motor activity to a specific end or listens to a voice describing this same motor activity. The observer's brain directly reflects the action being undertaken; the same cerebral areas are being fired in parallel in both subjects. The observer is mirroring the other person's behavior cerebrally.

The human brain has close to one hundred billion neurons. This cerebral galaxy features "mirror" neurons and "canonical" neurons. Our "canonical" neurons fire when we perform a specific activity, whereas our "mirror" neurons are only activated when someone else performs a motor activity or specifically describes in words a motor activity.

The first experiments were carried out on monkeys. When a monkey reaches out to grasp something, say a tennis ball, it activates a sequence of motor neurons in a specific part of the brain, which is perfectly normal. However, if the monkey simply watches another being—human or simian—reach out to grab a tennis ball, this fires the same sequence of motor neurons in the watching monkey as when it actively grasps something. In other words, when we observe others or listen to them, our brain mimics their actions and replicates the sequences, even, as far as language goes, replicating their words without necessarily pronouncing them.

In 2002, Evelyn Kohler discovered a distinct population of mirror neurons that she labeled "audiovisual" mirror neurons. Located in area F5 of the brain, they connect with Broca's area, the area of the cortex responsible for language. These neurons are activated both when a person observes effective action and in response to the sound of that action. The brain imagery of a person listening to a speech shows that the speech is silently being integrated, activating Broca's area: yet another effect of mirror neurons. The existence of these audiovisual mirror neurons has been verified through electroencephalography (EEG) and functional imaging MRI, techniques that give a visual display of blood flow variations in specific areas of the brain during motor activity.

To this day, only two cerebral networks have been discovered. One stimulates the frontoparietal mirror system located in the premotor cortex (Area 44 of Broca's area), the area responsible for language. The other is the limbic mirror system, located in the insula cortex and the limbic system. The mirror motor system is activated when we listen to and watch someone speaking.

This system is more complex in man than in monkeys. Mirror neurons are fired not only while observing someone else perform a precise motor activity but also when we listen to someone describing this activity.

In other words, as observers, our neuronal circuits are engaged exactly as if we were actively participating in the event: The observer is virtually engaged in the action observed.

In most cases, this is an automatic, unconscious epiphenomenon, which means that a double game is going on between the person speaking and the person listening: They are both at the same time actor and spectator. Currently, a multitude of extremely violent videogames on the market are popular with youngsters, hence the imperative need to fully assess the real scope of action of mirror neurons. These kids play out their videogames using the same verbal expressions as the characters in the game, the distinction between the virtual and the real becomes blurred, with potentially disastrous consequences for society.

The same personal involvement is operative when a child listens to its mother, or when students listen to their teacher, or the public listens to its idol. The common denominator here is their identification with the person talking, perforce associated with a degree of empathy. Emotions are one of the primary means by which we assess our interpersonal relationships, where we stand in relation to others and how we relate to ourselves.

Using functional MRI, Bruno Wicker established that when a person witnesses a patient expressing disgust, this activates the same neuronal sequence in both patient and observer. This is a shared neuronal reaction. It is almost a conditioned reflex. The observer isn't copying the patient and the patient isn't bidding the observer to react this way. This dual activity pattern, noted in the same area of the brain in both patient and observer, suggests that our capacity to experience and understand something that we aren't de facto actively engaging in stems from a vicarious experience enabled by both the brain and our hormones.

Your brain is full of surprises; mirror neurons are a system that links perception with motor activity. They reinforce the neuronal pathways of our motor brain. The more we activate one of these pathways, even through mere visualization, the stronger that pathway becomes and the easier it is to carry out the action it corresponds to. This no doubt is one of the reasons for the ever higher levels of tennis or golf achieved by these players. The move in these two sports is a real picture of the mirrors neurons influence. From childhood on, these players have visualized the matches of their idols hundreds of times over and appropriated their gestures. Similarly, in a political party, the leader often sets the tone through his or her voice, which party members reproduce, be it in terms of wording, of intonation, or of melody. All because mirror neurons have been stimulated.

In the case of our hearing, these mirror neurons already come into play in the womb. In the third month of pregnancy, the fetus begins to perceive sound, noises, music, and voices, especially its mother's voice, of course. The amniotic liquid modifies this acoustic mix. Low sounds are more truly sensed than high overtones, activating mirror neurons. The limbic mirror system makes possible the recognition of affective signals.

These neurons are enhanced in action. The limbic system is an active player in learning and memory processes. It enables us to link behavior and affect. The young infant is keen to please its mother; in response to her voice, to her lullaby, it seeks to share its sense of satisfaction with her.

Mirror neurons are involved in learning to speak, which requires developing the motor skills of the larynx, mouth, and tongue muscles. Mirror neurons forge links that escape all intellectual arbitration.

Studies carried out by Ionna Mari, Daniel Goleman, Gerald Hüther, and Inge Weser have thrown light on the different behaviors of the fetus. Man's progeny learns by spontaneously imitating what it sees and hears. Even before birth, the brain of a fetus registers a substantial catalogue that will feed its future memory bank of emotions, behaviors, actions, and, consequently, feelings.

One can easily picture the close ties that arise during a pregnancy between these two beings in symbiosis: a mother and her unborn child. Their two brains communicate constantly thanks to their mirror neurons. The mother sends information to the fetus every single instant. The voice is an unfinished symphony insofar as it continues to be written throughout its owner's life, but in the womb, the unborn child is literally in "sense surround," steeped in a sensory symphony in which the mother's voice and her bowel sounds prevail. Her voice forms the overture of the first symphonic poem of the voice of her unborn child, with its melodies, its prosodies, its rhythms.

Mirror neurons play an essential role in the life of the fetus. The wishes and longings of a mother reflect on the nervous system of her infant. Thanks to its plasticity, the brain of the young infant continues to develop until its 18th month, creating an emotional resonance in which empathy plays a primordial role. This information is the bedrock of every infant's existence as *Homo sapiens*, sowing seeds that will build, program, and sculpt many facets of its future life.

Mirror neurons have enabled us to decode scientifically the vocal and musical influence of the pregnant woman over her fetus, which is why I advise future mothers to listen to soft, harmonious music from the third month of pregnancy onward. The songs sung by the mother during her pregnancy and the music heard by the fetus will later have a soothing effect on the crying infant when it hears them again, enabling the infant to find peace and feel secure.

Epigenetics

At the start of the 21st century, we knew that the gene pool shared by *Homo sapiens* and chimpanzees differs by only 1%, in other words, 99% of our DNA is identical.

In fact, the genetic analysis of a *Homo sapiens* specimen around 100 years old reveals an DNA profile identical to that of the modern man. Thus, man's progress, evolution, characteristic communication aptitudes, voice, and richness of language impose the hypothesis of significant cultural transmission operating outside the scope of mere DNA. An astonishing study confirms this.

Two breeds of mice, A and B, were used for this experiment. Researchers took embryos from a female mouse belonging to Breed A, a breed with distinct characteristics, different from those of Breed B. They implanted the embryos in the uterus of a surrogate mother of Breed B. The conclusion is astounding: The young mice were found to have the qualities and behavior of the surrogate mother of Breed B and not of the genetic mother of Breed A. Therefore, at birth, the information pool of a newborn is not due solely to the genes of its father spermatozoids and mother egg but also to significantly and experiential learning it has integrated, appropriated, and inscribed in its cells during its time in the womb of the surrogate mice. How is this possible, which leads to a burning question regarding the impact of the voice: is it the mother's genetic voice or the human surrogate mother's voice that will have an influence and an effect on the baby?

Michael Meaney probes further with the following question: What happens during the first 12 hours of life ex utero? His research with mice, focusing on their first 12 hours after birth, is also impressive. He concluded from it that during this primal period, education can change the gene chemistry. The young mice that had been cared for by their mother—mice of Breed A—multiplied their neurons and their endurance to stress. The females later become caring and capable mothers. Meaney's conclusions suggest that all young children who have endured a difficult environment and angry voices may bear the consequences throughout their life in the form of a lesser resistance to stress.

The research findings of John Grabbe confirm it, "What matters is not only the genes we're born with, but also the way these genes express themselves. Our experiences change the expression of our genes, without changing our DNA. Our environment programs our genes and the way these will be activated."

Man has an exceptional aptitude for learning. It comes from the fact that at birth, we're not fully fashioned, not until 12 years old, but for some people like me, we are never fully fashioned!

Our gene pool is fixed through our DNA, but it continues to grow and to develop over time in its epigenetic expression. Thus, *Homo sapiens* has bountiful resources of adaptation to environmental conditions and influences.

Every new experience that the unborn child acquires through sensory, emotional, and mental perceptions enriches its cerebral neurons.

Homovocalis

Vocalis versus Erectus

Man made his appearance beside his primate cousins, the great apes, some seven million years ago. *Homo erectus* straightens up and turns into a biped. His brain develops considerably, including the area known as the neocortex, depository of language. The development of the cortex consecrates the brain as the orchestra leader of the voice. From hence on, nothing will ever be the same and no species from the animal kingdom will be able to equal man. The conditions indispensable for the birth of the human voice are soon met: verticality, the development of the resonance boxes of the vocal organ and the descent of the larynx in man's neck, from the first cervical vertebra down to its permanent position at the fifth vertebra.

Bipedalism made possible the verticalization of a fundamental element: the joint between the spine and the base of the skull, or occiput. This is also one of man's defining characteristics. It brings about a unique development of some of the cerebral areas, especially the development of language. The position of the spine in relation to the occiput is fundamental to the development of the brain; in monkeys, the first cervical vertebra is at a 120° angle to the skull, as against 90° in man.

A Noble Organ

The larynx is a wind and string instrument. It is an organ positioned in the throat between the pharynx and the trachea, a noble part of the vocal tract. It is designated as the organ of phonation. The two vocal cords are its dominant structure. An extraordinary scaffolding of muscles surrounds it, with membranes and cartilages remarkably supple.

This vocal entity captures its liveliness from the arteries and veins that irrigate it, its sensitivity and mobility from the nerves that control it, and its exceptional agility from the cerebral harmony that confers on it its identity as the vocal organ. Moreover, it plays a fundamental role in breathing and swallowing.

In the embryo, the pharyngolaryngeal crossroad begins to form after the third week of intrauterine life. At six weeks, the thyroid, cricoid, and arytenoid cartilages materialize. However, at this stage, the arytenoid cartilages and the cricoid are still fused together, as in other mammals. In the sixth month of intrauterine life, the larynx is now positioned as it is in chimpanzees. The epiglottis shortens, and the vocal space begins to take shape. Everything gradually falls into place during the 24 months following the baby's birth.

The ear, pilot of the voice, is one of the first organs of communication to be formed and solicited. From the fourth month of pregnancy, when the fetus begins to hear sounds, it joins the world of mankind, or more fittingly, the new world of *Homovocalis*. Therefore, its first contact with the outside world is through the voice. But, the fetus can't hear everything. In the maternal cocoon, that impressive matrix where life begins for the fetus, only low sounds are audible. High frequencies are absorbed by the amniotic fluid and thus don't reach the fetus.

The larynx lies much higher in the newborn baby than in the adult, close to the first cervical vertebras, as in chimpanzees. This allows the infant to breathe and swallow at the same time. In other words, to breastfeed for hours without one second off is possible! Why is it so? Because the baby breathes by its nose and the air goes directly to the trachea following the lateral part of the throat and the epiglottis, while the food goes through the mouth and directly to the esophagus in the middle part of the throat above the epiglottis. The larynx migrates down to the sixth cervical vertebra during the first two years, giving the infant time to build its resonance chamber, its "vocal cathedral" situated from the two vocal cords to the door of the voice: the lips. The toddler is then on board the team of *Homovocalis*, able to pronounce vowels and form words for the first time. Its "vocal space" is huge; the uvula no longer touches the epiglottis, which is really far, now until the age of 18 months, from the soft palate and the uvula. Note, if your child starts to speak at 10 months old, his/her larynx has already dropped to the sixth cervical vertebra. Well, from now on, the child could not breathe and swallow at the same time.

But is the female or male voice chromosomal—XX in the case of women, XY in the case of men—or hormonal? It is alchemy. Indeed, in both men and women, the larynx is hormonal dependent. It is the hormonal target of our voice. Does the gender of the voice depend on the XY or XX chromosomes or our sex hormones? The answer has been known since the 15th century: This is at the heart of the history of the castrati, males with with soprano vocal ranges produced by castration. The most famous was the celebrated Italian castrato singer, Farinelli. We will see this passionate "artificial" singularity later.

Women don't have an Adam's apple. When they reach puberty, their menstrual cycle begins and their voice changes under the influence of female hormones—progesterone and estrogen. Their voice drops, now three notes deeper than a child's.

The Phonation Apparatus: The Vocal Tract

Our vocal cords grow and change their structure right up to puberty. In a three-day-old infant, they measure 3 mm; at two weeks, they're 4 mm long; and at two months, 5 mm. In the five-year-old, they're 7 mm long and, at the dawn of puberty, 11 to

12 mm long. In adults, the hormonal influence is now maximal and the vocal cords are 17 to 20 mm long in women and 22 to 27 mm long in men.

We have two vocal cords. These are perpendicular to the trachea, and they form a horizontal V in the throat. The midpoint of the V is at the front, exactly level with the Adam's apple. The V doesn't stand for victory! It could, but in my opinion it stands for vitality, as these two cords are the trademark of humankind.

A key feature of the larynx, the vocal cords aren't, however, the only elements of the phonation apparatus, which also comprises the lungs and the mouth. The lungs provide energy for the voice. The air that is expelled from the lungs into the larynx allows speaking. We don't talk by inhaling air. Then, the vocal cords come together and vibrate. The resonance cavities—the pharynx, the soft palate, the mouth, and lips—enable articulated speech. In other words, when the lungs fill up with air as we breathe in, the vocal cords move apart. When we breathe out, the lungs deflate and the vocal cords join, producing voiced sound, be it spoken or sung. At the midpoint of the V, the vocal cords are in a fixed position, whereas the two branches of the V are able to close in, thanks to a joint that allows them to move toward each other or away from each other. Moreover, when we swallow, the vocal cords close, preventing any choking by blocking the entrance to the trachea. When we cough, the greater volume of air expelled causes them to close and open with force, as is the case when we sob.

The length of the vocal cords determines the frequency of the voice, while their tension determines both its pitch and its strength. However, the length of the cords isn't the only element that differentiates one voice from another. Genetic characteristics also come into play, as do other physiological features, for example, the size of the trachea or of the resonance cavities, such as the pharynx and the mouth. The bigger the resonators are, the deeper the sounds are produced and the richer will be their harmonics. The voice is a holistic rendering of the body. Each voice is unique, singular, and characteristic. It is fashioned by the resonance of sounds throughout the body, vibrating with our bones, of course, but also with our skin, mucosa, and various organs. The body is a cathedral and the larynx its pipe organ.

In the same way the violinist obtains the desired note by pinching a string so as to alter its tension and modify its length, we produce high tones vocally by lengthening the vocal cords, thereby thinning them, and low tones by shortening them, which fattens them. However, the degree of tension required to deliver a particular frequency depends on the diameter of the vocal cord. So, the length of the cord isn't the sole relevant factor in this process. The cord's thickness, its tension and its elasticity, which determines how fast the frequencies change, and therefore vocal vivacity, are all intimately linked.

For the violin to make a sound, the bow has to touch the string. As long as the bow hasn't moved across a string, the instrument will remain mute, since that contact is what produces the vibration. The same is true of the voice as the two vocal cords must make contact to produce a sound. When a vocal cord is paralyzed in abduction, no contact is possible and no sound is emitted. But if the paralyzed cord is positioned medially, in what is known as adduction, the mobile cord can still contact the paralyzed cord and thus produce vibrations. One of my patients, an operatic singer in London, sings despite her left vocal cord having become paralyzed because of breast cancer. Rehabilitation and her exceptional vocal technique made this feat possible.

Bear in mind that a vocal cord vibrates along its entire length. There is only one sinusoidal wave, and this physical characteristic is capital. Therefore, if you have a nodule or a polyp on a vocal cord, it may interfere with the contact between the two cords, but it won't prevent that contact, nor does it prevent the production of sound. If these "bumps" vibrate like the vocal cords, the voice may be stable. However, it can create a second vibratory knot that alters the voice by interfering with the frequencies, producing a raucous and husky voice. There are then two possible scenarios. Either this alteration is debilitating and requires surgery, or it doesn't unduly bother the patient. Sometimes, it may even be welcome if the hoarseness doesn't strain the cords, in which case it is best to leave it well alone. It becomes the person's vocal signature, a distinct voice imprint, as in the case of singers Ray Charles, Garou, or Joe Cocker. But in this case, the resonators play a fundamental role. Keen to demonstrate this, two researchers resorted to somewhat eccentric experiments.

In 1840, in Munich, Professor Pellisson extracted a string from his piano and fixed it to the wall of his bedroom between two nails. He pinched it, with no audible result. He then drilled a small hole in the wall at the level of the string. In the next room, he applied the piano's resonance box to the wall, over the small hole. He pinched the string again. This time it produced a clear, audible sound, distinctly recognizable as coming from a piano, which proves that the resonance box is a key element in sound propagation.

Another of his colleagues repeated the experiment, this time with a violin string. He moved the bow across it: It barely made a sound. Then he approached the body of a Stradivarius and a sublime sound was now produced.

If the A note produced by a violin or a piano is easily recognizable, the note isn't what enables one to recognize the instrument being played; rather, it is the harmonics generated by the resonance box that give a distinctive stamp to the original vibration, personalizing it. Thus, the shape of a music instrument, its texture, its internal structure, its geometry, and its elasticity all bring about the signature of its resonance. However incredible it may seem in the human voice instrument: the vocal tract!

Man's vocal cord presents analogies with a Stradivarius. The front plate of this remarkable *sui generis* violin is made of spruce and the back plate of maple. The meticulously precise distance between the two plates is mind-blowing. A wooden rod, called a sound-post, fits snugly between the two plates. This combination creates harmony and acts as a sound amplifier, giving the instrument its majestic voice. The efficacy of the resonance is enhanced by the fibrous nature of spruce, which helps to propagate the vibration. The human vocal cord presents a similar structure. Collagen and elastin fibers, linked by proteoglycan molecules, play a key role in the quality of the sound produced by the larynx. Nature has designed things in such a way that the mucous membrane of the vocal cord, which produces the vibration, is underlain with elements that embellish its resonance, delivering the first ever resonance box of the human voice.

In man, the resonance chambers fulfill the same amplifying role as they do in a violin, but the amplification produced is unique and unbeatable because the cavities are deformable rather than fixed. They're spread over four levels: the space above the vocal cords (the pharyngo-larynx); the pharyngeal neck above the cone-shaped larynx; then the buccal cavity, the nasal cavities, and finally the lips.

The buccal cavity deserves closer scrutiny. It houses the tongue, an indispensable ally of the voice thanks to its seventeen muscles. These exceptional muscles enable the mechanical production of vowels and, consequently, of articulated speech, for vowels are a fundamental component of the human voice. They result from changes in the length of our resonance chamber. Consonants are formed not by the vibration of the vocal cords, but by the resonators, during exhale. They are irregular sounds with scarce harmonics. Of variable length in speech, they're typically very brief when sung.

The anterior part of the tongue is mobile. The posterior part is fixed, or practically fixed, since a large part of it attaches to the hyoid bone. The tongue is the most mobile feature of this resonance box. When, upon exhalation, vibrations are transferred up through the various resonance boxes, the tongue can alter their pathway, widening or narrowing it in a thousand myriad ways. The two vocal cords produce the vibrations that convert themselves into articulated language when, '"dressed up"' as the voice, they arrive at our lips, forecourt of this vocal cathedral.

The voice draws its energy from our breathing. In adults, the inhale/exhale cycle is repeated seventeen times a minute. Our voice therefore is punctuated by the frequency of our breathing. When we speak, or sing, inhale is faster and shorter. It represents a mere 10% of the breathing cycle, the exhale taking up the remaining 90%.

Voiced sound is produced during exhale because of pressure exerted under the vocal cords. Mostly passive, exhale becomes active when we speak. It is then under our control, under our command. When it isn't, the vibration of our vocal cords is no longer in harmony with our breathing. This type of vocal abuse, which often arises in school teachers, and notably nursery school teachers, can lead to polyps, nodules, or keratosis forming on a vocal cord. Speech therapy is then imperative to relearn how to synchronisze the pneumophonic loop and thus restore harmony between the circulation of air to and from the lungs and the vocal cords vibrations.

In the neck, the laryngeal instrument is surrounded by numerous muscles, with the cervical vertebra at the back. An upright posture is inseparable from a beautiful voice. The backbone of this verticality is the bony structure made up by the spine and the cervical, dorsal, and lumbar vertebrae. It is the edifice around which muscular line forces are attached, like the sails and ropes that attach to the mast of a boat, and this enables the pneumophonic tube to be maximally efficient.

Cervical arthrosis can hamper the voice, as can any alteration of the dorsal or lumbar vertebrae. Osteopathy, a relatively soft complementary therapy, is often then a necessary course of action.

I usually tell my patients that if they take good care of their lungs, their voice will take good care of itself. Something all voice performers should heed if they haven't given up smoking, and that holds true for everybody. But these days, tobacco is no longer the only guilty party. Our voice must endure the consequences of a polluted environment, loaded with allergens.

When voice performers speak or sing, the vocal technique for delivering a sentence, prosody, or melody often involves short inhales that allow fast exhales. This constant to-ing and fro-ing of polluted air causes the vocal cords to dehydrate faster. Thus, the use of inhalers and aerosols, which have a salutary effect, should become an integral part of the way of life of all voice performers, who need to take care of their voice instrument like an athlete.

Measuring the Voice

Today, the new technologies of medical imagery allow this whole process to be filmed. I have the good fortune of having several of these machines in my office and I have adapted some of these. Modern technology allows me to directly view, at its actual velocity and at 4,000 images per second, the vocal cord vibration that bears witness to the existence of the voice. I know of few other dynamic scientific or clinical images that reflect so well the harmony of our own vibrations, vibrations that are so delicate, so fragile, and yet strong. It has the simplicity and the beauty of a beating heart. Such a sight makes the why and the how appear at times secondary; nevertheless, we still use a whole battery of units to measure vocal phenomena, the principal ones being listed here:

1. Pitch, low or high: This is the physical and acoustic measure in hertz, the male voice being 150 Hz, the female voice 210 Hz.

2. Vocal intensity, strong or weak: This is the decibel output, the normal voice having a 40- to 50-dB output (versus 119 dB for a lorry; our pain threshold is around 120 dB and crossing it can result in aero-otitis and tinnitus).

3. Rhythm, measured in seconds: It varies as a function of the variety of pauses, as in a musical score. The human voice has its own rhythm, which is a two-beat or three-beat tempo. The vocal rhythm requires pauses more than it requires silences. In an unprepared, spontaneous message, pauses are random, whereas in a prepared message, the pause is premeditated in order to stress a particular word—in effect a "rhetorical" pause. But the pause can also erect a virtual hierarchical barrier between two individuals.

Our Conductor of Our Voice

What is mind boggling is our ability to reproduce any note ad lib, be it a C3 or a D3. Each time, the vocal cords will return to the very tension, length, thickness, and elasticity required to produce that note and will adapt themselves to the right exhale pressure for the required vocal volume. And all this happens spontaneously. The human brain is wondrous indeed!

The brain is unique in more ways than one. First off, it is a topsy-turvy microcosm in which the right hemisphere controls the left side of the body and vice versa. Moreover, whereas throughout the body, from head to foot, the hard elements are protected—our bones are surrounded by muscle padding. The opposite is true of the brain as the skull protects and contains our mastermind, acting as an almost hermetic armor. Out of this protective box emerge, among other elements, 12 pairs of long cells, or nerves, whose role is to transfer information from the brain to the target organ. These pairs are perfectly synchronized. For example, the two seventh cranial nerves that innervate the face are perfectly symmetrical.

This mechanism is of a precision reminiscent of the great watchmakers, yet it harbors a rebel for the commander of the voice, the tenth cranial nerve. This pair does nothing like its fellow nerves! It alone has both a sensory and a motor function (it controls movements). It conveys to the brain how an action is felt and the sensitivity and excitability perceived by the target organ. It is the only nonsymmetrical pair. The 10th cranial nerve is different on its left and right sides, as far as the branch controlling the vocal cords is concerned. The left branch passes under the aortic arch before ascending in the neck, while the major nerve continues to wander down into the depths of our abdomen, since the 10th cranial nerve is much longer than others, despite being constituted of a single cell. On its path, it innervates the esophagus, the stomach, the liver and the viscera, and, partially, the heart and the lungs. Hence the challenge of finding a name for it; due to its perplexing itinerary, it was named the vagus nerve, or pneumogastric.

This 10th cranial nerve is the jack-of-all-trades of the nervous system: It responds to stress. It contracts the digestive tube and influences the production of saliva and gastric juices.

If the vibration of the vocal cords is passive and purely mechanical, the length of the vocal cord during phonation depends on the pneumogastric nerve. The master that rules over the larynx, our emotions, and our gastric reflux is therefore the pneumogastric nerve. The sensitivity of the larynx is also the pneumogastric nerve. The fact that a single nerve can convey contradictory information (both agonist and antagonist), as well as sensory information, is a unique feature of our organism. Should that nerve become diseased or sectioned, this would paralyze the vocal cords and alter the voice. The pneumogastric, called vagus or 10th nerve, enables the vocal cords to contract or relax. It controls their tension and their length and keeps them open during the inhale and exhale, and closed when we shout, cough, laugh, cry, vomit, swallow, and speak.

The vagus nerve, our stress nerve, controls gastric secretions and aggravates gastric reflux, with repercussions for the vocal cords. Voice performers could avoid the dysphonia problems they're frequently subject to by taking measures to ensure better lubrication of their vocal cords, a simple therapy entailing good food hygiene, steam inhalations using herbs such as thyme and rosemary, and an increasingly aggressive treatment of the allergic background.

A Few Key Words

The good health of the vocal mechanism, which allows one to avoid voice pathologies, incidents, or accidents, hinges on three key words: closure, vibration, and lubrication of the vocal cords.

Imagine your vocal cords as the palms of your hands. When you clap, the source of the sound is the contact between your hands. If you were to hold a ping-pong ball in the palm of one hand, instead of a clap, you would hear a dull sound. A polyp or a nodule is like that ping-pong ball. The vocal cords no longer come together. The voice then changes: As a matter of fact, the closure of the vocal cords produces the vibration. Their closure can also at times be affected when muscle fatigue inhibits closure; you can no longer "clap." This lack of muscle tone results in a husky voice. In other cases, the closure of the vocal cords may be impeded because a cord is paralyzed. The voice is reduced to a whisper.

Lubrication, in other words hydration, is just as paramount. If you set the tone to the standard A4 pitch, your vocal cords vibrate 440 times per second. Picture yourself rubbing your hands 440 times per second; they would heat up to a burning point. The same would happen with the mucous membrane of the vocal cords if it weren't permanently hydrated. A lack of hydration therefore debilitates the voice, which becomes hoarse, and can result in calluses and keratin plaques forming on a cord. These may require surgical intervention.

Our vocal cords suffer when overheated. A case in point is the dehydration of the entire pharynx and larynx, home to the vocal cord, when subjected to the acidity of gastric reflux.

Sometimes, only the vibration is impaired, as in the case of an infectious laryngitis or a fungus infection. It is your classical winter hoarseness.

Whatever the pathology, whatever the vocal problem, inevitably you find one of these three key words at the source of a dysphonia: closure, vibration, and lubrication of the vocal cords.

But other incidents can be due to emotion. Since the voice expresses our emotions, these incidents are frequent. Expressions such as "That concert left me speechless," "He took my breath away," and "I find that hard to swallow" are commonly heard. It's a fact that stage fright, the blight of voice performers, can paralyze the voice.

The color of the voice is modified by its environment and is affected as much by heat as by humidity. The alteration is most noticeable in certain harmonics, but it also affects sound velocity. Opera singers, whose art hinges on these phenomena, are all too aware of this. Singing in an empty theater doesn't give the same sound reproduction as does singing to a full house, the ambient air moist from the breath of 3,000 spectators. The resonance of the hall changes. The force of the different harmonics has changed. Greek amphitheaters show a perfect understanding of the importance of the "sound loop" created by the concave performance area of these temples of the human voice.

When the ambient temperature is 0°C/32°F, sound travels through the air at a speed of 330 m/984 ft. per second. (For the record, in pure oxygen, the speed is 317 m/1,040 ft. per second versus 1,300 m/4,265 ft. per second in helium. Therefore, if you speak straight after having inhaled some helium, you sound like Donald Duck, with a high-pitched, nasal voice and distorted harmonics.) The speed at which sound travels increases as the temperature rises, which is logical, given that a rise in temperature is nothing other than an increase in molecular agitation and that vibratory agitation is dependent on this same molecular agitation. In air, molecules are sparse. This isn't the case in water. Hence the speed of 1,400 m/4,593 ft. per second when sound travels in a liquid medium. The more humid the atmosphere, the more harmonics will be affected.

Moreover, a variety of parameters—temperature, degree of humidity, a background noise of 15 dB—can significantly alter a singer's audiophonatory feedback. The voice sounds different as a function of how the voice is absorbed by the ambient environment. The same occurs with the music instruments of an orchestra, which is why musicians retune their instrument just before the start of a concert when the house is full and after every intermission.

Just like an orchestra, the singer, the comedian, the lawyer, or the politician creates waves of vibration that are constantly changing and subject to their surroundings. The vocal power of voice performers also depends on how the concert hall reflects sound vibrations. Some venues are better suited than others. Certain theaters are dismal because the walls reflect sound back too quickly. If the vibrational return drops below 1/6th of a second, quite simply the intelligibility of dialogues is impaired. The reason being that our ear requires 1/6th of a second to distinguish between two phonemes. Happily, there is no shortage of acoustic temples, veritable vibrational lenses whose elliptic domes act as amplifiers for the harmonics of the human voice.

Singing, playing, pleading, and haranguing all require a suitably tailored vocal technique. Mastering the singing voice or the spoken voice imposes knowing your instrument well if it is to serve your emotional universe.

The instrument of the human voice is impressively precise. Getting to know it well and learning to understand it often helps to avoid unfortunate injuries. But the voice is exposed to dangers that one can't always guard against. That is when the mission of the Ear, Nose, and Throat (ENT) specialist or the speech pathologist comes into its own.

These Injured Voices

An Anthology

I recall Mr. R, a 60-year-old magistrate, who came to consult me because of vocal fatigue. After speaking for a mere 10 minutes, his voice became raspy. He complained also of not hearing well. His descriptions were theatrical as he mimed a judgment he was rendering in court. He bent fully forward, chin well up, head slightly turned to the left, pointing out that this was the position he must adopt when he listened to the counsel for the defense. His neck was strained, the muscles of his back maximally tense. All because he had to lean forward, due to impaired hearing on the left side, which has been bothering him for years. The excessive tension of the cervical muscles was causing severe and incapacitating muscle fatigue, which in turn distorted the muscles of the vocal cord. Hence his inability to speak easily for more than 10 minutes. In this instance, hearing, not the voice, was the issue. A hearing aid in his left ear sorted his problem out. The voice drives the ear.

Mrs. B., an opera singer of repute, was due to sing *La Traviata*, but in rehearsals, she noticed a loss of voice in the high notes. She came to consult me and despite a thorough videolaryngoscopic examination, I had no diagnosis. Yet videolaryngoscopy, and especially high-speed videolaryngoscopy at 4,000 frames per seconds, has made possible the discovery of a significant number of vocal pathologies that weren't detectable using Manuel García's mirror. In general, if I don't find anything, I don't tell my patients that nothing is wrong, I just tell them I can't see what the pathology is, which is completely different. This realistic attitude creates a climate of trust and leaves the door open for dialogue.

Thus, after a 20-minute discussion, this singer finally admitted having had a Botox injection to reduce wrinkling in her neck. But the injection affected the cricothyroid muscle in her neck, a muscle that enables one to transit into head voice, and her treble range was partially impaired. The only solution for her was to bear her misfortune patiently. She had to renounce her public performances for a month.

A Greek singer, I.R., consulted me for slight vocal fatigue and diminished performance at both extremes of the voice, though the treble range was more affected than the bass. Upon examining her, I detected nodules on the vocal cords. She was known and appreciated for her slightly husky voice. Her vocal cords vibrated normally. They came together satisfactorily. But a slight laryngeal dryness was noticeable. In her case, the only problem was acid reflux, which had to be addressed, but an operation should be avoided at all cost. Removing the nodules on her vocal cords could mean losing what gives her sensual and captivating voice all its charm.

After several months in musical shows, M.C.'s voice was broken. She could no longer sing. Upon examining her, I found hemorrhaging of the vocal cords, with a polyp. I insisted that her agent remove her immediately from the cast credits. I was not at all sure of saving her voice. The hematoma had impaired the vibration of the vocal cords and the polyp interfered with their closure. Moreover, the stress she experienced was causing acid reflux, impairing lubrication. In this case, of course, it was imperative that I operate. Restoring the spoken voice is one thing; restoring the singing voice quite another. Her reaction indicated she trusted me implicitly. "I have faith in you, I know you're going to cure me." Her attitude galvanized me and allowed me to consider an intervention using laser microsurgery, a combination of the laser as the surgical tool, the microscope, and video-surgery. This type of operation required some preparation. I first enjoined her to rest her larynx for a fortnight, as it was severely inflamed. In the meantime, I treated the acid reflux. D-Day arrived. I operated on her under general anesthetic, backed by the remarkable team I have been working with for years: same anesthetist, same nurse, same assistant. We discovered two polyps, with one hiding the other. Their laser ablation avoided any risk of bleeding. Then we removed the hematoma from the vocal cord. Postoperative enforced silence was essential for the next fortnight. Three months later, she was back on stage. Technology was on my side, but M.C.'s faith in me enhanced my surgical skills. My scalpel hand was guided by my experience but also by an "It Factor" that is a blend of art and science.

It was quite another scenario that brought S.-A.P. to my private practice. A 59-year-old barrister I've known for some time, his case illustrates all too well the vocal power that brings him to consult me. "My voice is playing up, I can no longer plead. Just thinking about taking the floor stresses me, I never know if I'm going to be able to plead. It haunts me. I can no longer concentrate on my arguments. For the past four months, my voice has become more and more hoarse. I was prescribed cortisone sprays, a treatment for allergic rhinitis, but nothing has helped. I still cough and almost suffocate now. My voice stills plays up, especially at the end of the day, and at night, I'm coughing more and more. I can't plead now. I'm so consumed by my voice problem that I can't focus on what I have to say. I'm no longer persuasive. I get the feeling it isn't me talking. The outcome is that for one month, I keep having to postpone my pleadings. My voice can no longer deliver my thinking." I interrupt him: "Why do you mean by no longer deliver your thinking?" He explains: "My thinking is killing me. It's too fast and my voice is too late. It's so revved up that my voice can't follow. My thoughts obsess me and my voice can't express them."

After this poignant confession, interrupted by fits of coughing and delivered in a broken, hoarse voice that at times was inaudible, what was I going to discover? The different tests showed he wasn't asthmatic. Yet his cough presented asthmatic symptoms. He suffered from a chronic rhinitis, with mucus running down the back of his throat, causing him to clear his throat frequently, with traumatic consequences for his voice. On balance, I found nothing of significance, except his impression that at mealtimes, he experienced a little acidity in his larynx. What

I saw seemed very benign; he could have spared himself four months of anguish. His vocal cords were mobile, but both were infected. His problem was a simple fungus infection! But there was more to it. What had allowed the mycosis to develop? Why had the persistent itchiness of the throat, symptomatic of a mycosis, only manifested a couple of months ago? He had another problem: gastric reflux, which antibiotics and cortisone couldn't resolve. The abdominal contractions provoked by the coughing had aggravated the reflux. I treated the mycosis and the gastric reflux and additionally prescribed an anxiolytic to treat his constant anxiety and stress. A fortnight later, the voice had recovered its normal function in the service of his intellect and, hence, its powers of persuasion, betwixt rhetoric and eloquence.

Mrs. B. C., a 32-year-old nursery school teacher, experienced a sudden violent pain on the right side of her neck, at the level of the larynx, while singing high notes with her class. She continued the rehearsal, but very quickly, her voice became deep before fading completely. She was obliged to put an end to the rehearsal. Worried, she burst into tears, concerned her vocal cords might be damaged.

I detected nothing abnormal when I palpated her neck. There was no evident sensitivity. However, the examination of the vocal cords was worrying. The right vocal cord, on the side where the pain manifested, moved normally but presented a hematoma, called in the jargon a subepithelial hematoma; in other words, a pocket of blood had formed under the epithelium of the vocal cord. Yet the cord vibrated. It wasn't inert. It remained supple. But the pocket of blood had changed the curvature of the cord, modified its density, and altered its balance and the vibrations. What happened here? She pointed out to me that before her menstrual period, her voice is often weak. She is then unable to use her voice normally. And four or five days before her menses, her legs feel heavy.

Conclusion: She suffers from vocal premenstrual syndrome. Examining her larynx, I detected micro-varicose veins on the cords. The veins are more fragile during the menses part of the menstrual cycle. Resting the voice completely while taking phlebotonics, magnesium, and an anti-inflammatory will fully restore her voice. In future, Mrs. B.C. will have to systematically take a tailored protocol of multivitamins, minerals, and phlebotonics 10 days a month, starting five days before her period.

L.M. consulted me, wanting to be free of stage fright. In my view, stage fright, stress, and dreading being on stage are essential to an artist's performance. Such emotional distress is something musicians, singers, comedians, and indeed all voice performers —conference speakers, teachers, lawyers, politicians, diplomats— apprehend. But in this regard, singers are the most vulnerable.

I explained to L.M. that when he takes the stage, he ceases to be L.M.; he becomes an artist who sings and communicates emotion. When talent prevails, stage fright vanishes. In certain cases, performers may need to take a beta-blocker but, happily, this is rarely necessary.

Céline Dion makes her voice dance. Her voice, timbre, and harmonics are to pop music what Maria Callas was to opera music. Her sincerity is reflected in her authentic singing. Both fragile and strong, she is full of emotion and endearing, both on and off stage.

A few years ago, at the start of a concert tour at the Colosseum of Caesar's Palace, in Las Vegas, Céline experienced some difficulty singing. A slight laryngitis was detected, but the examination of her larynx revealed nothing untoward. After discussions with her voice coach, Bill Riley, who was with her on tour at the Colosseum, the guilty party was revealed. The stage of the Colosseum was built with a slight 8-degree slope to ensure a good view for the spectators at the back of the hall. In trying to adapt herself to this slope, Céline was forced to adopt a bad posture. The forward bend of her upper body was damaging her vocal technique. In the long run, this could have had serious consequences for her voice and induce vocal forcing. You will recall the key role verticality plays in voice production, let alone in a vocal performance. Her coach ordered the stage to be made level and her problem was resolved. Céline recovered her vocal power in Las Vegas, on a stage tailored to her needs. A voice has to be observed holistically, in context, taking into account its environment; very often, a keen eye can avoid resorting to the scalpel.

In addition to voice injuries, the voice can suffer from natural lesions. The voice isn't exempt from aging. It can sometimes age prematurely in individuals who live in isolation and don't use their voice enough, bringing on an amyotrophy of the vocal cords. The laryngeal cartilages lose their suppleness and can become arthritic. Talking and communicating with others stimulates the voice and allows one to preserve its timbre. Illness and depression are two other factors that can prematurely age the voice, as can deafness. Indeed, the audiophonatory loop is essential to the preservation of the voice. Our teeth give away the age of our voice. Our mouth, exit gate for the voice, is bounded first by our teeth, then by our lips. The voice of a toothless, elderly person is deformed, and certain phonemes can no longer be pronounced. The lips stick to the gums and the tongue can no longer produce certain consonants. The solution lies in dental care and, if necessary, some type of prosthesis, such as implants.

The Basis of Good Vocal Health

I have for years tirelessly reminded my patients of the importance of vocal hygiene, giving them tips that may seem obvious, but are too often disregarded, notably before a vocal performance, or indeed, any time one needs to speak in public.

1. Mobile phones are very tiring for the voice. Why is that? Because there is no feedback of your own voice, people speak too loudly, with no retro-vocal control. When we speak on the phone, our voice is louder and pitched higher, which is more tiring. Long telephone conversations should therefore be avoided before a vocal performance. Something all of us have experienced at some time and that can be vexing: Two people chat at a nearby table, you can barely hear them, then one of them talks over the phone and your peace is shattered. It's a fact that our eardrums have no eyelids!

2. Avoid at all cost rooms with strong air-conditioning. Even worse is a sudden change of environment, going out into air that is too hot, too dry, or too humid, or going for a jog, just before a vocal performance. All this dries out the vocal cords.

3. Adopt a healthy, light diet. An overloaded digestive system becomes greedy for more oxygen. A heavy meal that sits like lead in the stomach will bring burps, belches, and regurgitations from the esophagus up to the larynx, or even acid reflux, which can alter the voice.

    Gastric reflux—stomach acid that moves up into the upper esophagus—is inflammatory for the esophagus and can burn the vocal cord. Our stomach can tolerate the high acidity of gastric fluids, and this enables us to digest what we ingest, but the esophagus can't, and the vocal cords even less so. Acid reflux can cause an inflammation of the vocal cords, as well as edemas or granulomas. It is also the most common cause of laryngitis and can bring about vocal fatigue, an urge to clear the throat, notably after a meal, also a tickly cough after a long telephone conversation. It is the origin of chronic coughs, improperly identified as being of nervous origin. When we stress, our stomach contracts and goes into spasm, increasing its secretion of hydrochloric acid and aggravating both our reflux and our stress. The stomach is producing more gastric acid than it needs. The reflux becomes endemic, inducing irritations that are often unpleasant, for both the sufferer and his or her immediate circle.

4. If we come out of a show, or a political meeting, or long pleadings, or a conference at which we have used our voice, and we proceed to a restaurant with a group of friends, we generally have to raise our voice in order to be heard at the table. It is a fact that in order to be heard, the voice needs to be 5 dB higher than the ambient noise. Hence the hematomas or micro-elongations of the vocal cord muscle that occur in voice performers, very rarely on stage, more as a consequence of celebrating their success. It is a bit like running a marathon, resting for 15 minutes, and then setting off for a

100-meter sprint. Inevitably, this invites injury, the more so if champagne, white wine, or rosé wines are drunk. These alcohols dry the vocal cords.

5. In an airplane, the engine noise is 70 dB. To be understood, we have to raise our voice to 80 dB. Aside from that, the lubrication of the vocal cords on board a plane is difficult due to an ambient hygrometry or humidity of the air of only 3%. This strains the voice, with the risk of small hematomas appearing on the vocal cord epithelium. Add a glass of champagne, and that dries out the vocal cord even more, and when we land, we've lost our voice. Which is why I strongly recommending that when you take a plane or a high-speed train, you drink water frequently, speak little, and avoid alcohol, unless it is red wine.

6. Sleeping or residing for some time in a house that is too humid, overheated, or too "dry" perturbs vocal performance.

7. The way we dress is also a factor. Avoid squeezing the lungs, wearing shirts with tight collars, putting pressure on the stomach and hence on the diaphragm, or wearing a belt that is too tight . . . opt for suspenders!

8. Two to three hours before a vocal performance, have a light meal of easy-to-digest food: complex starchy carbohydrates such as pasta, certain fruits (mangos, papayas, kiwis), or dry fruits. Give pepper steaks or cassoulets (a hearty French white bean and meat stew) a miss! Tea or coffee generally isn't a problem if they're drunk with moderation. One should drink frequently, but beware that hogging down half a liter of water in 20 seconds is likely to cause violent gastric dilatation and, inevitably, gastric reflux. Drink small quantities of water regularly, both before and during a vocal performance. It isn't unreasonable to have an energy drink as a supplement, for example, mixing half a glass of water with half a glass of an energy drink.

9. Dairy products, sauces, and cheese thicken phlegm and create mucus, inducing the urge to clear the throat and giving

the impression that something is stuck to the vocal cords, like chewing gum, a sensation that is heightened by gastric reflux. The voice breaks after 10 minutes.

Casein, which makes up 80% of the proteins in milk, is a major allergy trigger, behaving like glue on the pharyngolaryngeal walls. When casein-rich foods are consumed (milk, cheese, cream), the mucous membranes of the esophagus react by producing histamine (a substance stimulated by an allergen), which thickens the mucus. Which explains why many cases of dysphonia have both gastric reflux and an allergic background. I then prescribe a double treatment: an antihistamine and an antireflux. I should add that this pathology is more and more common due to the increase in pollution and our ever lower threshold of tolerance to allergens. Nowadays, close to one in two patients who consult me suffers from allergy, whereas 20 years ago, it was one in 10.

Anecdotally, Céline Dion followed my advice to the letter. When she gave birth to her twins, she stopped singing for several months and declared in an interview, "Having been warned off dairy products because they cause mucus in the throat that attacks the vocal cords, what bliss to finally be able to enjoy the dairy products I so love!"

10. White wines, rosé wines, and champagne should never be consumed before a vocal performance, due to the sulfite content of nearly all these wines. There are fewer sulfites in red wine, notably in Bordeaux wines, which don't seem to alter the voice. Even though modern beers mostly don't contain sulfites either, they do dry the vocal cords, due to the fact that they increase urination. The elimination of fluids induces a relative dehydration.

Certain individuals have an allergic reaction or, more precisely, an intolerance associated to an inflammatory reaction within half an hour of drinking a certain number of sulfites. The symptoms are a runny nose, sneezing, and possibly a headache. Close to 5% of asthma sufferers and individuals who are aspirin intolerant experience breathing difficulties in reaction to sulfites. These numbers should be kept in mind, given that 15% of singers are asthma sufferers!

11. Voice performers are athletes in their own right. For close to 25 years, I've been asking singers, comedians, and public speakers to do all sorts of exercise. This is essential if in this stressful world, one is to develop the abdominal muscles needed to eliminate aggressive toxins. The best sports are those that work the abdominal muscles and develop our respiratory rhythm, such as swimming and martial arts, sports that combine concentration and reflection. Such activities contribute to developing the full potential of the voice.

12. It is important to exercise the voice throughout one's life to avoid an atrophy of the vocal cord muscle and, in later years, arthritis of the joint on which the vocal cord inserts itself: the crico-arytenoid joint.

The Power of Vocal Seduction

Emotion Is a Mystery

Trying to pierce the mystery of vocal seduction is tantamount to taking the charm out of it. We align numbers and we align scientific, medical, and acoustic explanations, but fortunately, there is this inaccessible vibration, this ineffable charm. There is no point in owning a Stradivarius violin and knowing the secrets of its manufacture unless you are Yehudi Menuhin or Isaac Stern. Understanding the mechanism of the voice is essential; unveiling seduction belongs to a different register, that of emotion.

Beauty and emotion are intimately linked. Phono-surgery, the surgery of the voice, is a microsurgery in a class of its own. It is an emotional surgery. It acts upon the mechanics of the voice but also on the core of our being: our harmonious vibration. It is a microsurgery of emotion. Some of my patients, professional voice performers such as teachers, lawyers, journalists, singers, or comedians, talk about their work instrument as an instrument that needs to be "readjusted" or "retuned." Life's scars fashion their voice: Impaired, broken, or hoarse, their voice forges their personality, which far from being frozen, evolves over time, in accordance with their affective world.

The seductive power of the voice is unsuspected. There is no ideal standard of beauty for the voice, no Apollo or Venus of the voice. There would be no point in putting one forward!

In both men and women, the timbre of the voice, its musicality, its harmonics are an integral part of the personality. When we seduce with our voice, we create an inner radiance that engages, comforts, reassures, or galvanizes others.

Reducing the human voice, its charm, its personality, to the genes of the voice, to neurotransmitters, to the vocal cords, to Broca's area or to Wernicke's area, would be equivalent to describing a color painting by merely establishing the wavelength of its colors, red, green, or blue, with no sense of the harmony of the artwork. It would be like summing up Rodin, creator of the sculpture *The Thinker*, or Michelangelo, who undressed a block of marble to finally "tease" the statue of *Moses* out of it, as excellent technicians. Yet creation, in its strictest sense and unlike science, is none other than what is new, what has never existed before and cannot be replicated. "But science will be nothing without imagination," as Albert Einstein said.

About the voice, the creativity of the artist interpreting *Macbeth* by Shakespeare or Verdi's aria *La Traviata* indeed calls for a specific anatomical disposition and technique, but it also draws on the imaginary, on that indefinable something that is intangible and possibly divine: Do we not refer to the artist as a diva, a goddess?

A sonata by Beethoven can be analyzed as a physical phenomenon, on the basis of its sound vibrations. It can also be analyzed from a chemical, physiological, and psychological perspective, in terms of its impact on people, using different imagery techniques to observe the brain's reactions to the sonata. But the scientific dissection of a sonata doesn't make us like it. Only the seductiveness of the musical phrases counts. As Ludwick von

Beethoven used to say, "A false note is not important but playing without emotion is unforgivable." And that has nothing to do with science. Likewise, we can explain how the stars and the sun were formed, but when we behold the Milky Way, something else enraptures us, touches us, beguiles us, something that is fortunately beyond the realm of scientific analysis: pure emotion, a vibration that preserves all its mystery.

Seductiveness Is Still an Emotion

To seduce, the voice needs to be like music, and the melody and the words must provide clues or allow one to glimpse what is likely to reassure us, in the same way that a sequence of music allows us to infer what may follow. We're in known territory. But one false note and we're ill at ease, and the spell is broken. Should the voice rise, the crescendo needs to be done very progressively, without risking a sudden and unexpected high note that might cause some tension. Similarly, in a decrescendo, the voice needs to produce perfectly linked harmonics, with no aggressive break between two frequencies. Empathy and trust can only be established if the person being seduced is able to unconsciously anticipate what the seducer is going to say. This also holds true for the voice as projected in the media, by politicians and leaders.

In a subtext of seduction, two voices intermix, flirtatious, at times erotic. This vocal seduction necessarily involves acoustics, even when the exchange isn't face to face, as in the case of a telephone message or a radio broadcast.

One can fall in love with a voice. Certain patients have asked me to lend them the voice of Lauren Bacall or Marilyn Monroe, a voice that sounds alluring and sensual. Other patients may want a higher or a lower voice, as if they have become allergic to their own voice. However, their wish is rarely justifiable, unless they have a bitonal voice or a really irritating voice, a voice that rattles. As a phono surgeon, I can then try to improve their voice and make it a better "fit" for the physical body that houses it. Most of these patients are as unhappy with their voice as some others are with their body. I'm just the instrument maker of the voice, whereas they express themselves through this medium.

A seductive voice is sensuous, sometimes erotic, always emotional. On a first date, our voice is often tense; we speak too fast and our throat can sometimes be tight. Our pulse races, and our palms are sweaty. The reptilian brain is reacting. It has just released small hormonal molecules, such as adrenaline (hormones of stress), dopamine (hormone of desire), and oxytocin (the love hormone). The heart beats faster.

Attention to the Gorilla

During puberty, the voice draws from both hemispheres of the brain (the emotional right brain and the reasoning left brain); from the limbic system that houses our emotional life and includes the hippocampus, a structure closely associated with intelligibility and vocal perception; from the reptilian brain that controls impulses; and finally, from our hormones.

In nature, the gorilla puffs out his chest while hooting to show he is the dominant male, and the lion roars to keep his rivals at bay. And man? What does man do? Is there a relationship between physical strength and the voice?

There are vocal clues that in many cases allow one to evaluate the physical strength of a subject. Even on the phone, a voice can give some indication of the likely physique of the person on the other end of the phone. A telling study carried out in California by Aaron Sell, of Griffith University, in Santa Barbara, demonstrates this. A sample of 200 men from different cultural backgrounds—Americans, Bolivians, Argentinians, and Romanians—were first tested for muscle strength. They were then recorded pronouncing a simple sentence in their mother tongue, as the voice remains natural in one's mother tongue; it is our true voice, free of any extraneous accent, free of artifice. Female American students were then asked to listen to these recordings and to rate the physical strength of each speaker on a scale of one to seven. The result left no room for doubt. Whether or not the students understood the recording, they were able to form a fair idea of the physical strength of the man speaking just from the sound of his voice. It gave as fair an indication as if they had been shown a photo.

Aaron Sell interprets this result as a sort of heritage passed down to us from our distant ancestors. There was probably a time when from afar and at night, it must have been vital for men to be able to form an idea of the size of a possible enemy, just from the sound of their voice. The muscle mass of men being determined by their production of male hormones, its influence on the timbre of the voice is undeniable, as proven by their deeper voice. In a seduction scenario, the voice is an almost infallible source of information.

Take the mating call of the stag, in the autumn. The deeper the call, the greater the attraction for the hinds. In fact, the testosterone hormone thickens the stag's vocal cords, immediately producing a vocalization rich in very deep harmonics, which the hinds interpret as a sign of strength. Man is also a mammal with a reptilian brain; though he doesn't roar to attract a mate, his voice does provide information on his morphology.

One can notice a change in the voice of men and women who practice bodybuilding while taking steroid supplements and male hormone derivatives. Just like the biceps, the vocal cords are striated muscles that depend directly for their size on male hormones, which make the voice deeper. You may recall the female athletes from the former Eastern European countries: Being on steroids, they looked masculine and their muscles were anything but feminine. Their voices too had become masculine. On occasion, I've performed microsurgery on the vocal cords of some of these athletes to restore some femininity to their voice. The procedure consists of simply diminishing the volume of the vocal cord and, sometimes, its length (a procedure performed also on transsexual patients).

Though there are indeed links between testosterone, the muscles, and the timbre of the voice, reality is a little more complex. Low-pitch tones and a hoarse, gravelly voice don't necessarily go hand in hand with an athlete's build. In his experiment,

Aaron Sell didn't establish any systematic correlation between a deep voice and muscle strength.

The nuances of low notes depend on the presence of high notes. Very often, the beauty of a superb diamond is enhanced by its case; likewise, a deep voice that isn't offset by high-pitched frequencies that enhance it loses its power of seduction.

We know the voice has a mysterious component because it is what betrays our emotions; a few vocal notes suffice to unveil us.

Low notes resonate throughout the body. Testosterone, a hormone indispensable to the libido, deepens the voice, which no doubt explains why the impact of a voice is often a key factor in the seduction game of men and women. Don Giovanni is a baritone, his male voice embodies the seducer, the charmer, but it also intimates the risk of succumbing. In female singers, in the role of the alluring temptress, the low tones often contribute an erotic vibration.

A study by Robert E. Johnston, published in 2001, shows that women's attraction for deep voices is influenced by their menstrual cycle. In 2005, Dr. Puts recorded men with markedly deep voices, as well as men with a higher voice, whose recordings were tampered with to make their voices sound deep. The result was surprising: The men with an authentic deep voice were chosen for a long-term relationship, whereas those whose voice had been tampered with, to pretend having a deep voice, were chosen for a short-term relationship by women who were halfway through their menstrual cycle (when ovulating). Thus, not only does our ear identify the fundamental frequency that characterizes the pitch as low or high, but it also identifies harmonics, and these we can't fake!

In 2003, Sarah Collins and Caroline Missing delved into the question of the seductiveness of the female voice from a man's point of view. Men in the age range of 18 to 30 listened to women's voices in the same age range: The younger the voice, the more the men liked it.

It seems therefore that for both sexes, the seductiveness of a voice is linked to questions of sexual fertility. One could have surmised that women would be attracted to a higher male voice, such as tenors have, or that men would be attracted to a very high coloratura soprano voice in women. Such isn't the case! Both men and women are attracted by deep undertones: Testosterone therefore wins the day!

We know now that the voice depends on testosterone for its power of seduction. Indeed, for sexual desire to manifest in women, a concentration of testosterone of at least 150 µg is required, 250 µg being the required minimum in men. The ancestor of this hormone is the pheromone, the hormone of desire.

We find examples of seduction in bird behavior. Bird song is generally characteristic of male birds. An experiment was carried out with zebra finches. When testosterone was injected in female zebra finches, they could sing. But Robert Agate went further. This researcher from the University of California, Los Angeles noticed that some of these birds are male on the right side of the body and female on the left: on one side, a testicle and on the other, an ovary, which makes them both male and female, or gynandromorph. Their bird song is more powerful, their register wider than that of "simple" male birds. The right side of their brain is more developed than the left. This corresponds with the male side of the body. These observations confirm the important role of hormones in male birds. The gynandromorph zebra finch is the Farinelli (compared to the famous castrato) of the avian world.

Good Vibrations

In man, seduction isn't necessarily a preamble to mating or to procreation, but it always leads to a certain kind of pleasure, a preecstasy. Seduction presupposes having someone to seduce and the desire to seduce, but often, it also presupposes that the other person agrees to be seduced. The human voice is the vehicle of this transmitter-transceiver signal. It seduces by its very vibration. Its vibrations trigger and solicit certain stimuli, pheromones, and the secretion of sex hormones.

Emotion, seduction, and hormones: They're all linked. This vegetative reaction of our reptilian and limbic brains incites the hypothalamus to produce hormonal secretions. It is an impressive alchemy. Vocal vibrations suffice to release a flood of emotion, commingling beauty and seduction, eroticism, and ecstasy.

The voice, man's lyrical expression, is a reflection of our life, or more exactly of our lives, of our past, of our sufferings and joys.

The seductive power of the voice involves several criteria. Through certain vibratory reflexes, the voice stirs past impressions associated with a source of pleasure and well-being. Thus, the memory of the musicality of our mother's voice remains a key criterion all of one's life. Similarly, the melody someone hums will trigger the action of mirror neurons.

On the phone, one can "hear" the smile created by the bucco-pharyngeal resonance box. When we speak with empathy or while smiling, we contract our zygomatic muscles, the vocal cords shorten, the lips form a smile, and the eyebrows move away from each other. When we're being sarcastic, the voice is almost completely nasal, the pitch is low, the lips thicken, and the eyebrows arch in a circumflex accent.

A child's voice is fragile, inviting us to pay heed to it. A sad voice translates into a mellow, slow, low timbre almost devoid of nuances, a flat, broken, and plaintive voice. Surprise endows the voice with many harmonics. A boring voice generates insincere silences between words. The tone is fake. Some voices are quite the opposite of seductive. They can provoke aversion or repulsion: These are obsequious voices, overly languid, with totally artificial "enjambments." The angry voice is raised. The beggar's power is willful, his submissive, plaintive discourse, delivered in a weak and listless voice, creating feelings of guilt or compassion in others. Finally, the voice that signals a parting of ways, deception, or failure slows to three syllables per second instead of the usual eight characteristic of normal conversation; thus, there are numerous silences and the voice is apathetic. As for the sexy voice, it is easy to spot, humid, suave, with lower frequencies, a slower rhythm and sensual silences that leave one hanging on every word expectantly.

Each and every one of these voices has its own distinctive power. For example, laughter is contagious due to mirror neurons. A sensual voice increases the libido and the secretion of oxytocin, and a sad voice drives levels of pheromones down and increases the secretion of prolactin. Paradoxically, a voice that is too low is perceived as aggressive, whereas a high pitch—but not excessively high—voice comes across as friendly and empathetic. At the opera, is the tenor not the hero and the bass singer the bad guy?

The sensuality of the voice often derives from vibrational irregularities. In Germanic lore, the Lorelei had a bewitching voice that could be fatal. Ulysses was attracted to Sirens with their irresistible singing voice, power of the enchantress voice. The public speaker hypnotizes the crowd by communicating his singular vibration to his audience. Cyrano's lament under Roxane's balcony seduces the young woman by its vocal harmony, in which the words are notes. Yet Cyrano de Bergerac, despite his vocal seductiveness, is no Don Juan of the voice. Vocal philandering is a lure, as the voice can't lie for long. Mirror of the soul, it reveals our personality. It shines with the brightness of the sun, which, through the prism of the Self, distributes the colors of a rainbow, the nuances of which are specific to each of us.

Every Voice Has a History

With age, some voices become more reassuring, protective, and seductive. Others with advancing years sometimes need the help of a singing teacher, speech therapist, or laryngologist to recover their beauty and their charm.

The voice is a vibratory shield that battles against external aggressors. The resulting injuries and scars can sometimes lend a certain charm to the voice.

But it can sometimes change—become hoarse, metallic, monotonous, raspy, or dead—producing a loss of confidence.

Since the perfect voice doesn't exist, vocal imperfections are often the fountainhead from which seduction, charm, beauty, and attraction stem.

I listen to Louis Armstrong. His raspy, gravelly, damaged voice evokes for me all of the blues, his past, his resilience, but also the story of his kind, the history of the suffering of a whole population reduced into slavery. Clinically, his voice is pathological, but pathological as against what standard? I don't believe in the concept of a "normal" voice. A voice can come across as natural, particular, odd. It can be labeled pathological when a patient no longer recognizes his or her own voice, feels that it is broken, injured, or altered. The seductiveness, charm, and beauty of a voice are emotionally enriching for others.

I have more than once advised a patient against surgery if I thought her voice was authentic, sincere, and in harmony with who she was. Surgery should only be an option when the voice comes across as profoundly dissonant with its owner or when the owner perceives such a dissonance.

A striking example of this involves the case of a criminal lawyer with edemas on her vocal cords and a very deep, yet feminine voice. Her world was that of prison corridors. She defended big-time criminals. Her voice was an impressive asset, the timbre, between Edith Piaf and lower than Lauren Bacall with a strong personality. She wanted to change her voice to please her "man," as she referred to him. She told me, "I win all my cases, I am one of the best lawyers for criminals, they all know me in the penitentiaries but my man does not like my voice." After looking at her vocal cords, after having told her that there was no cancer but just an edema of the vocal cords, I answered, "Change your man, not your voice; your voice is your personality, your voice is you." She insisted on undergoing surgery. I had, however, refused to operate on her voice, and a colleague had stepped up. Her postoperative voice seemed superb, high pitched, extremely satisfactory. Anatomically and functionally it was great, but emotionally, it was a disaster. Yes, yet paradoxically, it had lost its charm and its sensuality. She therefore bitterly regretted the operation. Her "man" had broken off with her, no longer recognizing her, for she had changed "the face of her voice." This underscores the importance of our vocal signature. The lawyer's report back was dramatic: "I no longer recognize my voice. When I dream, I dream with my old voice, when I speak, I have the impression someone else is speaking, and I'm losing all my court cases. I've become schizophrenic through my voice!"

The Seduction of the Past

The voice and music are both universal; they exist in all cultures. Their strength, their sway has an undeniable link: They both stimulate our existence. The rhythm of a piece of music and the rhythm of a voice are fundamentals of the power they exert.

When we hear a regular beat, our feet unconsciously accompany it. We integrate that rhythm within fractions of seconds. If it changes, we follow suit immediately. These responses to rhythm are specific to *Homo sapiens,* but dolphins and parrots can also be taught them. The power of the voice is intimately tied to this: Acoustics are linked with movement in the central nervous system through motor neurons. This phenomenon of rhythmicity is well known in relation to Parkinson disease. Rehabilitation can be seriously improved through physiotherapy sessions in which the patient is made to walk and sing to the rhythm of music from his or her childhood.

Why would the neuronal condition of a patient be influenced by music from his or her childhood? The fact is that nostalgia has an exceptional power to unite and create empathy. The power of the voice when associated with music affects each and every one. Its power is moderated by the period it evokes and by the pleasure of the lost moment or the memories of a bygone adolescence.

A particular phase of life makes a person more open to being carried away and seduced. You invite someone you like to a restaurant; your voice is soft and sensual, you were careful to choose an establishment that plays background music that will remind your guest of a slice of his or her life, between the ages of 13 and 25. It is a moment of enchantment, seduction, and pleasure for both of you. Everything seems transfigured, the food, the atmosphere, the conversation. Harmony reigns, a mixture of camaraderie and desire, and your voice comes across as sympathetic, empathetic, and intimate. Is there a scientific explanation for this? That is what David Huron, professor at Ohio University, set out to study. When a subject in the 40 to 90 age range is asked to speak about his or her past, over 80% of the reminiscence focuses on the age range of 13 to 22.

The scientific explanation is multifactorial. When you're seduced by your partner, when you fall under the charm of his or her voice, when vocal eroticism prevails, oxytocin is secreted, the hormone implicated in our memory and social life. Simply being held in our partner's arms for more than 10 seconds (the time needed to stimulate oxytocin) while listening to music from her or his adolescence and hearing sweet words stimulates the production of this hormone and done, you are matched and harmonized. Its secretion varies as a function of age. It comes as no surprise that production is maximal between the ages of 12 and 22. At this age, desire is intense as we transition from adolescence to adulthood. Oxytocin is a major factor in social relations, in one's personal life, and in the desire to know desire. Hearing his or her voice while listening to music that triggers a sense of nostalgia will ipso facto release oxytocin.

Charisma

Is charisma, then, just a matter of oxytocin? When the power of the voice accedes to charisma, it once again eludes strictly scientific scrutiny, to rejoin the indescribable mystery of seduction.

A charismatic voice is a voice that resonates and keeps traveling through silence long after the last word has been pronounced, much like the sustain pedal on a piano, which results in sympathetic resonance and prolongs the last note played.

"What matters isn't what you say, but what the other perceives" is a basic rule of vocal charisma. Our energy, our inner strength, the sincerity of our mission, and our vision of life are the fount of charisma. Charisma allows one's light to shine forth. What we inspire in others by our words, by our empathy, by our need to give selflessly, that is the essence of charisma.

But I'm deeply convinced that each and every one detains this charisma, this divine gift, this personal magic, this inexplicable power. As Marianne Williamson so aptly says, "Who am I, to be brilliant, gorgeous, talented, fabulous? Actually, who are you not to be?"

CHAPTER 2

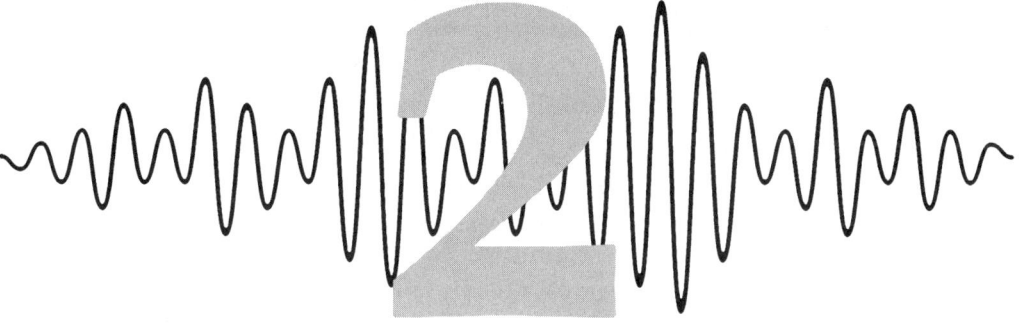

The Voices of Power

The Power of the Radio: Mars Attacks

On Sunday, October 30, at 8 p.m., the speaker announced, "The Columbia Broadcast System and its affiliated stations present Orson Welles and the Mercury Theatre live on the air in *'War of the Worlds,'* adapted from the novel by H. G. Wells."
At Orson Welles's request, this prime-time episode was to match with a Halloween dance, which surprised the station directors. Most of the listeners only tuned in to CBS after 8:15 p.m.; up until 8:12 p.m., they were listening to the highly popular ventriloquist, Edgar Bergen, and his puppet Charlie McCarthy, on NBC. Welles was well aware that the audience wouldn't have heard the announcement at the start of the episode and would therefore take the drama of *War of the Worlds* at face value. While the orchestra of Ramon Raquello was on the air live that evening, playing in the Meridian Hall of the Park Hotel Plaza, the music was suddenly interrupted by a news flash announcing that

Professor Farrell, of the Mount Jenning Observatory, had identified explosions on planet Mars. The rest is history. Orson Welles went beyond the adaptation of *War of the Worlds*; he updated it by going on the air as a news reporter. His text was written like a last-minute information, not like yet another chronicle.

The scenario had been meticulously rehearsed, with the news announcements interrupting the media, the Halloween show, rather than the other way around. Welles put silences to good effect and invoked the testimony of listeners, who were taken in. He adopted a somber, tragic tone. His voice was low, captivating, and uncharacteristically calm. The mystery was amplified by his voice timbre, which invoked a reflex of fear.

That evening is now legendary. The very next day, supposed scenes of panic and massive manifestations throughout the United States made front-page news. A tell-tale sign of the reigning hysteria: witnesses reported having experienced physical symptoms, such as gas emanations from the Martians and the heat emanating from their weapons.

Which elements enabled Orson Welles to make his hoax seem credible?

Above all, he changed his voice: the tone, the language used, and his self-assurance contrasted with his earlier bland and innocuous episodes he used to present before. That night, the actor excelled, scoring and marking far beyond his expectations. Bear in mind that Orson Welles was only 23 when he concocted this fake radio broadcast, not to say this acoustic mirage. Orson Welles was born on May 6, 1915, in Kenosha, Wisconsin. His childhood was one steeped in the world of puppet shows, makeup kits, and the magician's paraphernalia. These three alchemical ingredients laid the groundwork for Orson Welles's future accomplishments. At the age of 10, this budding illusionist of the voice played *King Lear*, disguised as an old man. Aged 17, he made his stage début, in Dublin. Aged 20, he arrived in New York and created his own company, the Mercury Theatre, which ran aground. In order to recover financially, Welles agreed to work for CBS. The station asked him for a series of 1-hour episodes, to be broadcast once a week, on Sunday evenings. The first four episodes were a complete flop, and the audience ratings couldn't have been worse. That was when he came forward with his now-famous adaptation, to be aired on the night of a Halloween celebration. Overnight, Welles became an international celebrity and Hollywood opened wide its doors to him: in 1941, he directed a masterpiece, *Citizen Kane*.

That evening wouldn't have had the same impact without the collaboration of experts, scientists who agreed to come on the air to comment on the events and maintained a periodic radio presence throughout the episode. If you want a lie to be credible, add a grain of truth, with the endorsement of scientists and a sincere, persuasive, and low voice. On that night of October 30, 1938, Orson Welles returned to the magician roots of his childhood to become the grandmaster of the "make-believe voice" as a ventriloquist that he was also.

The media impact of the voice, which triggered the phenomenon we call a rumor, was able to generate collective fear by creating doubt the world over as to the frontier between legend and reality. And when the legend exceeds reality, we prefer to believe in the legend.

The Power of Speech Therapy: The King Stutters

It was only in 2010 that most people learned through a remarkable film, *The King's Speech*, that the King of England, George VI, stuttered. The film explains that due to his handicapping stammer, Prince Albert had never envisaged mounting the throne, the more so since his older brother, King Edward VIII, had been next in line. But the latter abdicated in 1936 to marry a divorced American, Wallis Simpson. And thus "Bertie" became George VI, in 1937. Henceforth, his stuttering was no longer a personal matter but a state affair. He had to learn to express himself without the slightest hesitation. The voice of a ruler, of the person in power, can't afford any debility and must never invite mockery. Having suffered from this disorder since the age of eight, and that had progressively worsened, Prince Albert had always feared public appearances. His closing speech at the British Empire Exhibition at Wembley, on October 31, 1925, when he was 29, was an ordeal for him and painful for his audience. This distressing episode led him to hire Lionel Logue, an Australian speech therapist, who remained his therapist throughout his life. Logue was convinced, and rightly so, that this elocution problem could be resolved.

Until then, the radio had been little used by people in power. During millennia, kings, emperors, and pharaohs hadn't needed their voice to assert the symbolic authority of their word. By right, their legitimacy was hereditary, not popular, and they enjoyed supreme authority over their subjects thanks to their privileged closeness to God. They represented their power through imagery: an official portrait, a signature or a seal at the bottom of a decree, an effigy on a coin. This mute, silent representation allowed an element of mystery to prevail. In the 9th century, Louis II could get away with being king and stammering, but in the 20th century, this seemed impossible. The more so since George VI faced a terrible adversary, Adolf Hitler, and his appalling, disgusting, and orgasmic vociferations. He just had to bark and his audience transformed itself into a pack of rabid dogs. The individual ceased to exist. Hitler used his voice to manipulate others, be it when perched on a bistro table in the 1920s, or later, facing a microphone, in a stadium where he hypnotized thousands of people.

George VI faced a difficult task. Yet the British sovereign wasn't short on bravery, nor did finding the right words fail him; he just lacked elocution, vocal fluidity, and rhythm in his speech, all essential when speaking on the radio. Thanks to the efforts of both Lionel Logue and his patient, something extraordinary happened. George VI delivered his speech in a voice that may seem slow and at times chanting, but overall, behooved the dramatic turn of events. He had made haste slowly; like all stutterers, he had played with the silences. England would join in the war; he had been convincing in the aftermath of a fierce internal battle, the intensity of which only he was privy to. With great difficulty, he worked at sculpting his voice like clay, crafting the words every second of his speech. And a miracle took place. The history of the human voice is full of these miracles.

When I listen to George VI, to his silences, his dry voice and his breathiness, I also hear his anguish and his hopes, his tenacity, his patience, his victory over himself. Through the interplay of mirror neurons, that voice awakens in me not only my own anguish but also my hopes. I embrace this voice, I become a part of the sovereign's voice, and I am ready to follow the head of the armed forces almost blindly.

TV and the Power of the Voice: An Emotional Amplifier

In time, it was inevitable that the speech pathologist I had become would take an interest in the voices of the people who lead us and attempt to discover the root of their specificity. I laid down my stethoscope and, like a detective, delved into the archives of the INA, the French National Audiovisual Institute, which were kindly made available to me. With eyes closed, I listened to a great many speeches by political figures, both past and present. I also viewed very attentively the preelectoral televised debates, "scrutinizing" the voices and all their variations, especially the winner's, whose voice would one day govern. I pulled together data that included the rational sphere, the spiritual sphere, the instinctive sphere, and the emotional sphere. What I refer to as "the body language of the voice" fascinated me, since the body also talks!

But before seeing what lessons this methodical profiling has to offer, I would like to share some observations that became evident to me. In political rallies, the speaker addresses the crowd directly, and on the small screen, each viewer is targeted. Television is an awesome emotional amplifier. It gives equal exposure to someone genuine and to someone devious, does it not? **But when it unmasks a cheat, it has no compunction shooting the person down in front of viewers as a gladiator in the arena.** A look, the lifting of an eyebrow, a movement of the shoulder or of the hand can be dead giveaways during an eloquent rhetoric. Seduction alone doesn't cut it; you need to deliver a message that is congruent with your attitude and be in earnest.

The political speech is carried by exhale. It requires a rhythm and a technique that politicians need to master if they're to forget their voice and focus only on their message. Their persuasive skill and pertinent improvisations are the hallmark of great orators. Unfortunately, in our societies drowned out by voices, often the message of the political speech seems secondary and politicians are remembered only for their mannerisms and the color of their tie. The paradox is that in this world of the Word, we seem to evolve in a world of mime. We're submerged by so many multiple voices that we end up listening to none. We would like to take refuge in silence, but silence can't find its place in the deluge of words. The journalist for the eight o'clock news has to string the news together without a breather, at the expense of the intelligibility of the broadcast. Political information is reduced to a series of clips or a "voice snapshot." The same applies with respect to the radio. The station head is constantly gesturing to those behind their microphone, urging them to speed things up. Their delivery is therefore no longer natural. Gone are the days of attentive listening, now replaced by frenetic communication of the message. We need to find time again to listen to that inner vibration, and we must trust our inner truth and communicate it, so that our voice may be heard and escape the media frenzy that is threatening our acoustic world. That is in fact why televised debates are so popular. They offer their audience the opportunity to get onto the same wavelength as the debaters, these modern-day gladiators. You are the judges, they are the battlers. Your decision will kill them or make them alive.

The First Duel

We're in 1974. Valéry Giscard d'Estaing and François Mitterrand, between two rounds of the presidential election, confront each other in a live televised duel, followed by 25 million viewers.

This kind of confrontation has long been standard practice in the United States, but in France, this is a first. Everything has to be invented from scratch. The rules that were defined then still apply today: random draw of the first speaker, strict enforcement of equal time for each speaker, and validation by the campaign teams of the debate's producer, facilitators, and decor. Broadcast on all three television channels, this debate, facilitated by journalists Michèle Cotta and Jean Boissonnat, made history.

Valéry Giscard d'Estaing understands the situation perfectly. He is spontaneous, comes across as sincere, and, more important, shows a lot of empathy. Giscard is filmed up close, hands joined under his chin, as if in prayer. He has registered that in a presidential election, more so than in any other election, it is the man who gets chosen, not a project, hence, in my opinion, the almost religious pose he adopts. The moment is solemn. The words he is about to pronounce will be determining, and contrary to expectation, politics are no longer the subject; sentiments are: "First, I'm always shocked and hurt when someone appropriates the control of the heart. You do not, Monsieur Mitterrand, have the control of the heart! You do not . . . I have a heart, just like yours, that beats at its own rhythm and is truly mine. You do not have the control of the heart. And don't talk to the French people in that offensive manner." The register is low, no high notes at the end of a sentence, the tone firm, comforting, never condescending, always respectful. He knows how to reassure. From this long litany, a single word emerges, loud and clear: Mitterrand. Giscard is heard: Mitterrand is being hurtful, not just toward his adversary, but through him, toward all French people, whom Giscard is trying to bring together around him, as if saying to them, "Rally yourselves to my beating heart!" Empathy is as its peak. Mitterrand, who is off-screen, mumbles a timid, echo-like "Of course," which sounds like an admission of defeat. I should point out that back then, François Mitterrand considered the camera "a black eye" that petrified him. He would say that to win, one has to be genuine, but that it is very difficult to be genuine when faced with a bevy of machines, journalists, and people of all ilk. In any event, victory befell the candidate who had known how to use these two factors: a scathing yet respectful reply and an empathetic speech. Only later did François Mitterrand come to realize that in an election, public opinion counts for less than the public's affection. From this standpoint, this debate is a classical case study, as empathy and instincts play a key role in it.

Empathy

The German philosopher Robert Vischer created the term "empathy" in 1873. *Einfühlung* means felt from the inside. Empathy is a notion that signifies the "comprehension" of the feelings and emotions of others. The term is different from "sympathy," which presupposes a dialogue, an exchange. Sympathy can be gratuitous and generous, and it gives protagonists a chance of agreement. Of variable intensity, it is an expression of compassion. Sympathy is vibrational and outward directed.

Empathy has frequently been investigated with functional magnetic resonance imaging (MRI). When we see others in painful situations that have an accidental cause, it activates the neuronal circuits of the somatic-sensory map associated with physical pain. This neuronal network involves several parts of our brain: the insula, the cortex, and the gray matter. It would seem that this sensory-somatic resonance mechanism between others, relatively primitive on the evolutionary plane, and us is already in place at birth. This mechanism plays a critical role in the development of empathy and moral reasoning. It allows us to share in the distress of others without being judgmental. It also allows us to inhibit aggressive behavior.

This feature probably appeals to our primitive or reptilian brain, seat of our reflexes and impulses. Indeed, a captivating study has shown that rats who learn to press a lever for food will give up eating if they realize that by their action, another rat will receive an electric shock. They would rather die of hunger. We too have this mechanism that allows us to share in the distress of others, and we modulate it subconsciously. Various factors can inhibit it or increase it. These factors can be social, ethnic, political, or religious.

We're not far off the phenomenon of mirror neurons. When we watch a football match or a tennis match, we replicate the same neuronal circuit, provided of course we love the sport, as emotion plays a fundamental role here. The spectator lives all the points of the match. The adrenaline rush is at its peak. The link between perception and action is crucial. The voice produces comparable effects on the individual and on the group. And those who lead us use this same impressive power.

A crowd behaves like a single brain, the single neuron, YOU, of which would be the individual crowd members; stimulated by the leader's voice, these neurons, all the "you," behave like mirror neurons. Such is the power of the voice on a crowd. Individuals no longer exist as such; they merge with the group.

The group anesthetizes the individual consciousness. They project themselves as one into the discourse; they *drink in* the words. More exactly, they integrate these words and appropriate them. When they agree with the politician, in effect they're in agreement with themselves.

Taming the TV

France had not known a presidential election by universal suffrage since the Second Republic and the election of Louis Napoleon. Universal suffrage was brought back under the Fifth Republic, during the two-tour elections of December 5 and 19, 1965, which opposed General de Gaulle and Mitterrand. In 1958, an electoral college had elected General de Gaulle president.

This institutional upheaval coincides with a technical revolution: the arrival of television in domestic households, even though in the 1960s, only seven million French owned one. For the first time, thanks to television, electors were invited into the political arena. At first, politicians were reticent, not least General de Gaulle, who only made two appearances on "the box," to intimate that France must choose between him and chaos: "Should the strong and massive adherence of citizens enjoin me to remain in office, the future of the new Republic would definitely be ensured. Otherwise, no one can doubt its immediate collapse."

In 1965, Charles de Gaulle instigated a remarkable democratic revolution by accepting the terms of a televised electoral campaign open to all parties and that guaranteed all candidates strict equality of speaking time.

In this new context, the general-candidate sought almost exclusively the sympathy of his pairs, World War II veterans, thus neglecting those who never knew the Liberation and overlooking in his addresses the lively postwar youngsters who weren't impressed by all these medals. He thereby cut himself off from a part of France. Unexpectedly, he found himself in a hung vote with François Mitterrand, a politician who couldn't boast a glorious past in the Resistance, despite being a methuselah of the Fourth Republic. Indeed, he never referred to 1945 in his speeches. He managed to gain the support of left-wing sympathizers, showing his capacity to accept opinions that didn't quite fit his. De Gaulle quickly understood the need for a new strategy and, between two tours, granted television interviews to the journalist Michel Droit, who would be put to task again twice, in both cases at a critical and sensitive time for the general: in May 1968 and in April 1969, on the eve of the referendum that would lead to his early retirement.

In December 1965, de Gaulle had realized that the new battles ahead would be fought on the small black and white screen that robbed the speaker of the vibrations of a crowd, of emotional feedback, of the capacity to improvise according to the energy of the audience.

The first interview was significant. It covered Europe and agriculture, two subjects that bear no relation to anything military. De Gaulle adopted the stance of a veteran soldier. The term "veteran" is loaded, underlining the fact that his military past was most definitely history. The ploy was successful. The general became the presidential candidate, a man of the 1960s. Some of his utterances have since become proverbial and attest to this metamorphosis: "The housewife wants progress, but she doesn't want a mess!" "The Left party isn't France! The Right party isn't France!"

He became the providential man of the new republic, but more than that. He spoke not in his name but in the name of France. He was elected with over 55.2% of voices. And Mitterrand was consecrated "the man of the Left party."

The second tour of the 1969 campaign may not be etched in people's memory, but it is particularly significant and fascinating when analyzed in relation to the almost caricature aspect of the power of the voice.

The French had a choice between the former prime minister, Georges Pompidou, and the interim president, Alain Poher. The Poher/Pompidou duel may have raised a smile or two due to its alliteration, as well as the specter of having to choose between two products of a same brand, but it didn't stir any enthusiasm. The 1969 election was the only one in which the voter turnout was better in the first tour than in the second tour. Jacques Duclos, the candidate for the communist party, back then one of the leading opposition parties, exhorted voters not to opt for six of one, half a dozen of the other, which voting for one or the other of the candidates would have amounted to, given the similarity of their ideology.

Yet their voices, or more exactly the ways they used them, set them worlds apart. Alain Poher preferred to address the French without anyone to contradict him. Alone facing to the camera, he embodied the past, the drama actor reciting his text, and what a text it was! Filmed close up, he came across as smug. Although born in 1909—he was 20 years younger than de Gaulle—he seemed to belong to the last century. He spoke like a drama actor, with a theatrical timber. The tone was peremptory. He was the man of yesteryear.

He began his allocution with "I had promised you chaos would be avoided": He wasn't even yesterday's man; he was a man of times long gone! The rest is in a similar vein. When finally the camera pans out, it is to show the interim president extracting from his inside pocket a leaflet criticizing his own program, and which he started to read, his glasses tucked up his forehead: "I give you six reasons for not voting Poher, my opponent." In so doing, he is lending the leaflet credibility, because putting things into words gives them substance. He puts his glasses back on, folds the leaflet, and digs himself deeper into his speech: "My turn now to recall the past," he says. With Poher, devising tomorrow's policy is once again all about taking a step back. To make things worse, he then makes another blunder by addressing Pompidou directly, which makes Pompidou look good. "I, for one, didn't have the honor of being the Prime Minister of General de Gaulle." If you needed a good counterexample of a vocal performance, Alain Poher could be your man. He is glued to his text, reading it with application, without the slightest trace of affect, empathy, or hope, and even less of any dream.

Not only did Pompidou choose to be interviewed, but he chose to be interviewed by no less than three journalists, two women (Annick Beauchamp and Rose Vincent) and a man (Christian Bernadac), in a cozy lounge setting with leather armchairs and a coffee table. At the outset, Pompidou invited his rival to "turn to the future . . . , like all French people." Right away, the musty Poher, his opponent, was sent back to his fossil past. Pompidou expressed himself in simple terms, in a serious, rather monotonous voice; the tone conversational, quite at ease. This vocal attitude, which concords with the decor of the interview set, is all it takes to turn the situation around. Despite having been in power for five years, one vocal conjuring trick makes Pompidou the man of the future, despite his voice being firmly in the present. But more is needed. To be sure to win the election, he needs another interview. When Jacqueline Baudrier asks him what his impressions will be if he is elected president, Pompidou is pensive, then answers with an anecdote. When a Roman general was victorious, he was carried triumphantly. But the person at his side carrying his laurel crown was there to remind him that he was but a man and that his victory belonged to all and sundry.

Thanks to this anecdote, Pompidou introduces empathy. If tomorrow's man makes reforms, it will be for the general good.

More than any reform project, more than any answer, more than any personal anecdote, this reference says it all. Pompidou's past as a graduate from the prestigious Ecole Normale Supérieure and as a scholar—de Gaulle had selected him when on the lookout for such a graduate with writing skills—and the notion that culture must be at the service of others, must be shared. You have to grant it to Pompidou. He was the first to have understood the secret to winning elections in televised interviews.

Maybe his love of the arts had something to do with that. The ultimate artist is the one who keeps up with his time and may even be ahead of his time if he is a visionary. As far as I know, Georges Pompidou was the only president to have exercised the privilege of his position to visit museums, at any time of day or night. Art, or at least the love of art, is a powerful expression of empathy, which is why it is a good omen when a presidential candidate is sensitive to art. In my view, art is timeless, comingling present and future, and a head of state who hasn't understood that culture is the marrow of a nation has understood nothing, as it is culture, not war, that endures.

The best example is still François Mitterrand: together with Jack Lang, who was a worthy power behind the throne. He instigated an event that is the perfect embodiment of empathy, an event at which emotion is at its peak: "La Fête de la Musique," which became an annual, worldwide summer music festival that should happen every year on June 21st. This was decided in October 1981. Jack Lang, Minister of Culture, appointed Maurice Fleuret to the position of Director of Music and Dance. Maurice Fleuret applied his reflections on musical practice and his evolution and laid the foundations for a new conception: "Music will be everywhere and the concert nowhere!" It evokes a "revolution" in the field of music, which tends to bring together all the music—without hierarchy of genre or origin—in a common search for what he calls "a sound liberation, a drunkenness, a vertigo that are more authentic, more intimate, more eloquent than art." Disparaged, snubbed, and criticized, nevertheless all over France, it remains an undeniable showcase moment of sharing.

Every victory François Mitterrand has had bears witness to his perfect understanding of empathy.

He used it in a most unusual way, as by nature he wasn't inclined to be generous. He played with irony, using it to gain sympathy, to the detriment of his rivals. In the midst of the 1988 debate that opposed him to Jacques Chirac, who was the prime minister:

> Mitterrand: "I watched you for two years and you give me a very bad example. But I do not want to commit myself more. I do not make any particular comment on how you express yourself; you have the right to do so. I continue to call you 'Prime Minister' since that is how I called you for two years and that you are. Well, as Prime Minister, I noticed that you had very real qualities but not those of impartiality and justice in the conduct of the state."
>
> Chirac: "Let me tell you that tonight I am not the Prime Minister and you are not the President of the Republic, we are two equal candidates who submit to the judgment of the French, the only one who counts. You will allow me to call you 'Monsieur Mitterrand.'"
>
> Mitterrand: "But you are absolutely right, Prime Minister."

The president had just inflicted on his adversary a brilliant verbal slap in the face, all the more crushing because it left no room for rebuttal.

Mitterrand's last reply—for it is indeed one—provoked surprise. Moreover, the greatness of the political phrases to the astonishment, which it provoked, was recognized. "As in a fable, the sentence must be rather short, unexpected and spontaneous. It must upset the mindset of those in front," explained Adrien Rivierre, who knew perfectly the recipe for this success. With this small sentence, Mitterrand recalled that he was the only one to incarnate "the presidential authority." His voice was calm, with low frequencies and a perfect rhythm.

The words become the foam on the voice wave.

Winning Voices

Not all presidents are aesthetes, far from it. My primary intention in using these examples was to analyze the different forms through which some of these presidents expressed empathy in their talks. But there are different forms of expression. Aside from its aesthetic form (Pompidou, Mitterrand), there is also the heroic form (de Gaulle, Giscard d'Estaing) of men who go to battle, for real or symbolically, and make the offer of self-sacrifice for their country. This being said, to be in this category, you don't have to have served in the military or have a noble title (e.g., Nicholas Sarkozy, who loves a good sparring match and challenges). A dueling man, he promised the French people he would be their champion, a modern-day champion at that, on the security front and on the economy front, both policeman and accountant.

In 2007, the final battle was no longer a man's prerogative. The debate between the two rounds is very instructive on this point. Despite having a softer voice, Ségolène Royal each time was the one who went on the offensive, finally losing her composure. The discussion centered on the treatment of diabled children in school: "I think we've reached the height of political immorality . . . and I'm very angry. —Calm down, retorts Nicholas Sarkozy. —No, I won't calm down." And now the verbal slap in the face: "I don't think you're elevating the dignity of the political debate by calling me a liar . . . I don't question your sincerity, Madam, don't question my morality." At this point, Sarkozy no longer looked at his adversary. He knew he had the upper hand. His voice remained calm, with low harmonics, while Ségolène Royal ended her sentences on a high pitch that provoked an irritation in the listener.

As for the Sarkozy-Hollande duel in 2012, the same parameters prevailed: "I want to be a president who first and foremost respects the French and has a high regard for them. A president who doesn't want to be the president of everything, head of everything, yet at the end of the day, responsible for nothing." François Hollande set the tone, one of empathy and sharing. His timbre was low and calm. He detected a crack and stepped into the breach. He followed on with an improvised monologue lasting over three minutes, consisting of an anaphora repeated 15 times: "If I'm elected president of the Republic. . . . "

Whether they use it as artists or as soldiers, our presidents use vocal empathy. Those who haven't known how to endorse one of these two suits have always been beaten. All except Jacques Chirac. Admittedly, Chirac is a died-in-the-blue aesthete, but nothing in his discourse betrays his love of the arts. This is a man whose passions are discreet. Despite listening to his discourses over and over, I detect little empathy in them, yet in a small group, it shines through richly. The media ramp can sometimes be ruthless. But it is true that this head of state is a silversmith in another domain: sympathy.

When Hands Talk?

The archives of these debates offer us the privilege of allowing us to see the gestures that are an integral part of vocal power. Hands also talk. When President Mitterrand rubbed his hands together, it was his way of installing a climate of exchange.

The position of the hands, if too high or too low, can be upsetting for the person opposite. The voice then has a negative impact. The hands should be positioned somewhere between the top of the speaker's chest and the belly button. They need to be visible and expressive if they're to support the discourse without interfering with it.

An open palm, facing upward, beckons to others; it is an element that unites, a call to assemble, to adhere to the discourse. All children between the ages of two and five open their palms up toward you when they speak to you. Conversely, a downward-facing palm that flashes at you is a defensive posture. If this gesture accompanies the words, "what do you think," in effect it means the speaker has already made up his or her mind and won't be open to what you have to say. However, the same gesture, when accompanying the words, "Hang on, let me finish!" is perfectly justified. When you clasp your hands together in front of you, you're creating a barrier between you and the other person, taking your verbal distance from him or her. The hands then offer the protection of a virtual pulpit. Conversely, a person who speaks with palms facing upward, extending them toward the other, is signaling openness and verbal generosity, which invites empathy.

Why is this "hand body language" so important? Every gesture an orator makes when discoursing should be in harmony with the language of his or her hands; otherwise, there is a disconnection between what the audience sees and what it hears. He or she then becomes the forger of his or her own voice. Likewise, looking the other person in the eye is fundamental, as the eyes reveal the truth of your words.

The Intentions of an Address

Reviewing these audiovisual archives led me to identify five key intentions of voices in power: to assert oneself, to install a climate of trust, to share information, to convince, and to touch the heart of others.

The First Intention: To Assert Oneself

That is the strength of politicians who have no pretense and are self-confident enough to be themselves. Conversely, for those who depend wholly on others for their self-image, their voice is a lifeline. Since they only exist through the ears of others, they talk nonstop, because they don't exist if they're not talking. They become hostage to their acoustic mirror, in the same way that Narcissus was hostage to his reflection.

The Second Intention: To Install a Climate of Trust

In a political rally, the orator allows for breaks in the discourse, winning the audience over through humor and challenges, seeking to create complicity with the audience. Another way of installing a climate of trust is to speak in a low voice, re-creating conditions that foster intimacy, something that the television and the radio proscribe. In these instances, the voice encourages complicity with the auditors. You're confiding with yourself on the doorstep of a friend without intruding in his or her home.

The Third Intention: To Share Information

Every discourse contains a message, but how can you be sure it has been received? Rigor is required. The objective is to ensure that the person opposite, the spectator or the militant, remembers the talk. Jargon is your enemy. You want to be understood by all and sundry. In any message you're delivering, the meaning of your words counts, of course, but the impact you have stems from the power of your voice. A voice that becomes low and deep, enriched by silences that are the muted words, becomes the power of persuasion.

The Fourth Intention: To Convince

You're angling to get others to adopt an opinion, or to change their opinion, knowing that vocal impact isn't just about projecting yourself onto others, but also its appropriation by others once it has been heard. The voice no longer belongs solely or completely to the one trying to be convincing. Nurtured by its environment, by the vibrations in space, the power of the voice can't develop without implicating the person listening, who is vibrating and transmuting it in his or her emotional filter. A warm, almost intimate voice is able to vary the tone, alternately endearing, poignant, or pathetic.

I can remember very precisely a conversation I had with Robert Badinter some years ago. He was the justice ministry. It was at the end of my consultation, at 7 p.m. I was lucky to be able, after the medical problem resolved, to talk with this remarkable man. I was in favor of the death penalty for certain acts I consider unforgivable. Within half an hour, he did change my way of thinking. Admittedly, Robert Badinter, an exceptional man, had significant arguments. But beyond his arguments, the tone of his voice, his sincerity, and his verve rang true. The alchemy between his conviction and his emotions transcended his words. How did he convince me? He just pointed out that as an individual, he can understand "the revenge mind" of you against somebody, but as a man taking care of the collectivity and not the individual, it is not acceptable that a community gives death penalty.

The Fifth Intention: To Touch the Heart of Others

Emotion is an indispensable component of the four previous intentions if these are to blossom. Without emotion, even the most exceptional arguments will fall flat. An emotional charge is therefore necessary if these intentions are to have any sway in a discourse. Deprived of emotion or feeling, the reasoning mind expresses only sterile concepts; no sooner pronounced, they cease to exist. Therefore, emotion has to be created, accentuated, or toned down. Take fear, for example. A high, fast, quavering, almost breathless voice, practically bereft of silences, accentuates fear. Conversely, a deeper, almost confidential voice, of which the volume button is perfectly mastered and turned down low, minimizes fear. That voice is reassuring; its vocal body language must be in harmony with the discourse held. Emotion can't transpire if the speech isn't punctuated by breaks. To create emotion, all the nuances of the vocal palette have to be used. Therein lies the genius of the actor.

The Voices of Leaders, Singular Voices

The heroic voice of Churchill or de Gaulle, Hitler's hysterical voice, the reassuring voice of Chirac or Mitterrand, Bill Clinton's husky voice, and Obama's wisdom voice, not to mention the voices of Gandhi or Martin Luther King Jr., these are proof enough that no standard magical formula applies to the voice of leadership, and that is fortunate.

One can still try to understand the power, mastery, and charm of these voices and attempt to establish the vocal imprint of a leader. How do leaders impose their voice on a crowd and to what extent do their voices answer to particular codes or follow fashions? Would such a scrutiny not present an opportunity to distill out of it a "library" of politicians' voices, classified according to the urges they stir in the masses?

Salvador Dali's Orange-Colored Lamp

Perhaps the best place to start is an anecdote I was told by a very dear friend, a close friend of Salvador Dali's.

Mad genius, eccentric, artist, and alchemist surfing between chaos and harmony, reason and madness, the vibrations of colors and the dazzle of lights, Salvador Dali developed a bizarre spectacle in his studio to accompany his creative work. He listened to records but wanted more than just sound. Various lamps strewn about the floor would go on and off in step with the acoustic vibrations. The sound waves appropriated the vibratory space. Each lamp emitted a different color that would light up in accordance with the harmonics, frequencies, and pitch of the voice. Thus, the lamp filaments emitted light vibrations in reaction to the acoustic vibrations. Each frequency, each note corresponded to a specific color. A festival of light and sound, in typical Dali style! In this psychedelic setting wafted the acoustic waves of Brahms, Beethoven, or La Callas, as well as certain speeches or poems Dali enjoyed listening to. Oddly enough, one particular orange-colored lamp at the back of the studio would never light up. Until the day Dali decided to put on one of Hitler's harangues. Surprise, the orange-colored lamp lit up, reacting to an ultra-high pitch that only the "Führer's piercing timbre" had stirred and that had not appeared in any sonata. It may be these same vibrations that had been able to hypnotize an entire population and galvanize crowds.

Hitler progressively raised the pitch of his voice with every new sentence, whether or not it posed a question. The result was that each sentence seemed to end with a bang or a gunshot, in that overly high-pitched tone that had caused the orange lamp to light up, almost, it seems to me, revealing its existence. At the outset, he doesn't speak loudly; at any rate, his sound volume is much lower than in any rock concert, but then he raises his voice higher and higher. There is also a change in pace; he talks faster and faster.

Before being a string of words, every discourse is first and foremost music to our ears and heart. It appeals to our hearing, to our emotional world, before appealing to our reasoning.

Thus, three successive and insuperable stages can be identified: The orator addresses himself first to our hearing (a mere fraction of a second, in the order of one-fifteenth of a second, suffices to integrate the message), then to our reptilian brain (the brain that reacts to impulses and primary reflexes), and, lastly, to our reason. We hear, we feel, we understand. In my eyes, this chain of information is key for understanding the voice.

Where alchemists sought to transform lead into gold, the ear for its part discreetly pulls off the feat of transforming a sound first into liquid, then into a chemical substance. The message passes through the outer ear, then the middle ear, and, finally, the inner ear. When in the middle ear, it can be minimized by a small muscle lodged at the door of the inner ear, known as the stapedius muscle. When sound reaches it, it contracts, withholds the sound, and then transmits the vibration after a latency of 40 milliseconds. The inner ear transforms the mechanical message into a chemical message.

More than words, it is the musicality of the voice that rules us, with its sounds, its frequencies, and its rhythm and musical orientation. All orators are pretty much aware of this. "Music before all else," Paul Verlaine, a poet of the 19th century, was fond of saying. How right that is, and yet this evidence is often only integrated on a subconscious level. Those who lead us captivate us and invite us to follow them. Sounds, not words, make this happen. Voice is first heard and then experienced emotionally by the reptilian brain; words are there simply to give direction and are processed by the cortex. Emotion turns into affect, gateway to the world of reason.

Words guide us on the foam of the voice wave that imposes the emotional tide.

I as in Icarus or the Virtue of Obedience

You may recall the film *I as in Icarus* (*I comme Icare*), a film by Henri Verneuil, with Yves Montand. This 1979 film pretty much transposed Kennedy's assassination to an imaginary country. Among its other merits, it features an experiment on obedience to authority figures, an experiment that really took place in the United States between 1960 and 1963, conducted by the American psychologist Stanley Milgram. The aim of the experiment was to understand the limits of obedience: how far would someone go to obey a figure of authority, be it scientific or military, as in the film.

A student, in fact a comedian hired for the purposes of the experiment, strapped to a chair, receives fake electric shocks every time he makes a mistake memorizing words fed to him by a teacher who is also an accomplice. Increasingly strong electric shocks are administered by the test subject, who has no idea the shocks aren't real. Soon, the student is writhing in pain and begging for the experiment to stop. In the film as in the actual test, the conclusion is chilling: The subject waited until 175 volts had been administered before manifesting any reticence.

Thus, we learn that "63% of subjects are obedient, in other words they totally go along with the principle of the experiment and apply up to 450 volts . . . which means that in a civilized, democratic and liberal country, two-thirds of the population are likely to carry out any order given by a figure of authority." In this instance, the voice was justified by the scientific basis of the experiment, allowing the Cartesian mind, almost sovereign, to become the voice of power.

To give legitimacy to the abuses they perpetrate and pretend they've taken over the reins of power peacefully, without resorting to physical violence, tyrants act as if verbal violence doesn't exist and can't lead to bona fide psychic rape. Tyrants stir up the primary reflexes of the masses in order to prevail over them. Observing the reactions of live beings to any type of stimulation can help us better understand the reactions to certain discourses, to certain words or intonations.

If we're to understand the power of the voice, we need to get back to Pavlov. I see food, I prepare to eat it; before I've even brought the food to my mouth, my brain has decrypted the information: I'm salivating. In the same way and by analogy, I hear an order given by a figure of authority; my first reflex is to obey that order. On the salivary front, it's a reflex; in other words, an adaptation by the organism to a given situation, a reaction in which the central nervous system (CNS) transmits and coordinates the excitation stimuli and their effects. The CNS here has a decision-making role. This is a remote reaction. Seeing something triggers an internal biological response. It is therefore a conditioned response that stimulated the salivary glands. The reflex salivation only occurs after repetitive learning; this conditioned reflex is therefore very different from the innate or automatic responses of the newly born, like the gripping reflex.

The word, the command, or the voice is only able to subordinate if the other's psyche has been conditioned, is in distress, or is physiologically debilitated. Resistance to subordination is conditioned by a sociocultural context that prevents the bedding down of primary conditioned reflexes. Education empowers criticism of the discourse. Ignorance, lack of education, and lack of experience make people easy targets, over which control can easily be gained.

The voice of power is channeled through various vocal modalities. Back to Pavlov. One of his experiments involved separating a litter of puppies into two groups; both groups were taught conditioned reflexes. The puppies in the first group were free to roam; in the second group, the puppies were caged for 2 years. The second group less easily integrated than the first group. This "caged group" presented greater sensitivity to sounds of excitement and to vocal stimuli. These dogs were fearful, trembling at the slightest noise, and the voice had a big impact on them. The freedom experienced by the puppies that had experienced multiple stimulations due to their freedom to roam made them slower to respond to a conditioned reflex.

As far as the power of the voice goes, we're all Pavlovian dogs. No need for sweet talk or careful wording; only the tone counts. If you use a friendly and playful voice to say to a dog, "You're going to be beaten, whipped and left without food for eight days," the dog will come to you without distrust. Conversely, if you promise a thousand caresses and treats but in an aggressive and menacing voice, the dog will immediately take off. So the timbre of the voice is key. When sad, it becomes pathetic; too joyful, it becomes flippant and loses credibility; too high, it becomes irritating. So what, then, is the ideal voice for a leader? Does it exist?

Is There an Algorithm for the Voice of Leaders?

Four Instincts, Four Behaviors

Leaders need to know how to be liked. They protect the crowd, more specifically, the individual amid the crowd. This individual behaves like a child, is irresponsible, follows the group, is immature, and is manipulated; in a crowd, an emotional cement forms, and the individual is no longer fearful and accepts to be led and to obey. Indeed, the fighting instinct, the survival instinct, the parental instinct—the leader protects us—and the pleasure instinct are the four principal characteristics of our leaders' voices. These criteria are remarkably analyzed by Tchakhotine in his book *Le Viol des foules: The Rape of the Masses by Political Propaganda*, published in 1939. The author shows how reason is bypassed and how the psychic mechanism of the reptilian brain and of the prefrontal cortex interconnects. On the basis of Pavlov's reflex theory, Tchakhotine develops a line of thought according to which leadership draws from four major instincts characteristic of man:

> A1 is the first instinct: the fighting instinct.
>
> It feeds on the urge to fight death, to avoid danger. It calls on the survival instinct. Fear, anguish, depression, but also bravery or enthusiasm can constitute the stock-in-trade of the voices in power.

A2 is the second instinct: the feeding instinct.

It feeds the urge to act for the survival of the species, also called the feeding instinct. It highlights economic advantage and financial profit. It acts by performing a balancing act between misery and poverty, dreams and hopes. If the wording is right, it can convince the hottest dissidents.

A3 is the third instinct: the sexual instinct.

More limited and more specific, it calls on the instinct for self-reproduction and therefore for self-preservation. This instinct has two fundamental components: primitive components that provoke erotic excitation and sublimated components that thrive on music, singing, beautiful women, artists, and models.

A4 is the fourth instinct: the parental or protective instinct.

The leader's voice subjects the crowd to one or several of these four primary instincts. They have a nigh subconscious impact. The individual members of a crowd react without any real cognizance.

But these four instincts seem not to be the sole constituents in the algorithm of the voices in power.

I found four other behavioral criteria. If these four varieties of discourses are also taken into account, the result is impressive.

Indeed, this powerful conviction displayed by leaders also draws on four other behavioral criteria that seem to me to be indispensable and complementary in relation to the four instincts:

B1 is the first behavior, mystical or religious.

B2 is the second behavior, a rallying one (for the group, using a warfaring or military approach).

B3, the third behavior, is the expertise criterion (through reasoning and scientific analysis).

B4 is the fourth, charisma, which is fundamental.

But let us pause here and try to profile our politicians and leaders against these eight criteria. All of them display at least six of the eight criteria. Below six, they seem to have little chance of becoming a leader, a politician, or a CEO. For example, referring to the letters A and B and numbers attributed above to each instinct and behavior, we find:

François Mitterrand: A1 A2 A3 A4 B1 B2 B3 B4: exhibits eight criteria.

Martin Luther King Jr.: A1 A2 A4 B1 B3 B4: six criteria.

Jacques Chirac: A1 A2 A3 A4 B1 B2 B3: seven criteria.

John Fitzgerald Kennedy: A1 A2 A3 A4 B1 B2 B3 B4: eight criteria.

Bill Clinton: A1 A2 A3 A4 B1 B2 B3 B4: eight criteria.

Barack Obama: A1 A2 A3 A4 B1 B3 B4: seven criteria.

Gandhi: A1 A2 A4 B1 B2 (he maintained that one cannot preach nonviolence and also be a warrior) B4: six criteria.

It is up to you to add to this list.

The Group Anesthetizes the Conscience of Its Individual Members and Hypertrophies Their Emotional World

Hence their uncritical ear and blind obedience ("It's not me, it's the group"). Hitler only existed and posed a threat thanks to the might of the group he had put in motion.

Besides the voice of the politician, of the leader or dictator, symbols such as a logo, a song, a rallying cry, or a specific salute are primary elements of propaganda. They not only constitute signs that enable individual group members to recognize other members but also are very effective for conditioning followers, exculpating in advance any possible excesses. "It wasn't me, it's the group. The boss told me to do it." The symbol marks its territory; it compels with no explanation needed. It illustrates the code of the group; it belongs to *this* group, and the individual is exploited. Indeed, when individuals are questioned on their own for an opinion survey, they don't have this group mentality, and they don't give in to their primary instincts. They don't have that right. But in the group, in this so-called anonymous crowd, reasoning no longer prevails; emotion does, the more so when members are driven by fear of insecurity, threats from other groups, or the material and feeding instinct ("They're going to take all we have," "We have to defend ourselves," etc.). The voice of hatred is aggressive; the voice of fear is defensive. Symbols appeal to the emotional child at the core of every individual. The voice differs according to what drives it, whether it's the will to fight, desire, paternalism, or religion, and yet all of these voices lead us.

An orator of Jean-Marie Le Pen's impressive stature is able to surf the collective instinct, reclaim the crowd's hysteria, channel it and direct it, and alternate violence and aggression in his discourse and in the power of his voice. He mobilizes emotions and fosters a climate of fear through his pseudo "expert" analysis and by claiming allegiance to a group using his own distinctive code (these rhythms so typical of the orator's voice).

The voice of Obama addresses itself to the minority instinct, which overlaps with the feeding instinct or the material instinct, as well as the parental instinct, a mechanism that also appeals to a man's pride. As part of a group, the individual can accomplish anything: "Yes we can."

In the same way, Martin Luther King Jr.'s voice refers back to the parental instinct, associated with the spiritual instinct. "I have a dream . . . my children."

In a different register, the pope also seeks to reassure: "Don't be afraid." Here, too, the parental instinct comes through loud and clear.

To govern a group, a leader must create the conditions for members' allegiance to a cause, to a collective logic that they can identify with. His voice must resonate, solicit images that are familiar and reassuring, present a melody as well as silences that raise questions to which the audience must expect answers, and be eager to be comforted and reassured. Orators must remember to insert a few good words here and there in their discourse, a little irony that relaxes the atmosphere and produces laughter, which is the best way to forge the cohesion of a crowd, giving it a feeling of relative complicity. The voice becomes the cement that is the bedrock of its power.

A Singular Case: General de Gaulle

The rhythm of the voice's breath and melody is as important as the signifier. General de Gaulle's emotional energy was particular. The rhythm of his sentences coalesced with the magic of his words, forming an impressive alchemy, always on the brink of tragedy, of fear and of confidence, of paternalism and indisputable authority. In my opinion, de Gaulle is an outstanding textbook case. In June 1940, he stirred up the fighting instinct of the French. He belabored them, he diatribed against France's enemy. The tone is military, punctuated, unadorned, a tone that doesn't invite any comeback. De Gaulle had been entrusted with a mission by his country: "La France libre." In Paris, in June 1944, the orator spoke in the deep voice of a tragedian: "Paris! Paris outraged! Paris broken! Paris martyrized! But Paris liberated!" These words are now so famous that their tone is almost forgotten, firm, assured, the tone of a people who no longer have to fear for their survival. It's a prime example of the feeding instinct, also of the sexual instinct, the dominant male asserting his leadership. Over the years, how did this military and informative voice fare? The voice of the general became the voice of the president of a free nation. The voice evolved, became in time paternal, protective, with compassion (the family instinct): "Je vous ai compris!" (I did understand you!). De Gaulle took ownership of the collective emotion. Then the voice became almost tragic, in true Malraux style, as the president announced that at his age, he would never undertake the career of a dictator. He wanted to reassure this new generation of French who hadn't known the war and who doubted their own country or, more precisely, the regulations and laws of France. Once more, the general showed himself to be an exceptional strategist, a strategist not of the battlefields, but of his voice in the media.

In the France of May 1968 student revolution, in the Latin Quarter of Paris, was the scene of confrontations and clashes between the authorities and students. The protests spread progressively to all economic sectors of the country. France was paralyzed from May 13 onward. On May 24, de Gaulle pronounced an address on French television, a popular expression back then. At this time, France had only one channel! Seated at his desk, he looked somber and responsible. People listened and criticized but didn't really pay attention to his comments and warnings: "For nearly thirty years now, events on several important occasions have obliged me to assume responsibility for getting this country to take its destiny in hand, in order to prevent others from doing so against its wishes. I'm prepared to do that yet again. But this time, especially this time, I need, that's right, I need the French people to speak up and express their wishes.... A referendum is the most direct and democratic way forward." Thus, a man in his 50s talked on television of France's "revolutionary" backdrop. He had little impact, and the protests continued. But the statesman, the strategist in him was stirred. On May 29, General de Gaulle disappeared without explanation for an unknown destination. Consternation! Even the prime minister had no idea where "Le General" might have been. Speculation was rife. In Germany, in Baden-Baden, General Massu received de Gaulle. Was he thinking of resigning? Was he looking to secure the support of the armed forces? No sooner back in Paris the next day, he gave another address on television, but his tone was firm in the presidential speech he gave. The "president General" was impressive, or rather his voice was, during his discourse on May 30, 1968. At the time, I was a student at the faculty of medicine in Paris, and I can remember it as if it were yesterday. It was 4 p.m. The general spoke on television, but the screen was blank. His voice replaced the image. The general was invisible. We listened to him; his voice was firm, without a trace of hesitation. Its timbre, rhythm, and musicality are engraved in my memory: "Men and women of France, as the holder of the legitimacy of the nation and of the Republic, I have over the past 24 hours considered every eventuality, without exception, which would allow me to maintain that legitimacy. I have made my resolutions. In the present circumstances, I will not step down . . . I am today dissolving the National Assembly. As for the general elections, these will be held within the period provided for under the Constitution, unless the intention is to gag all French people to prevent them from expressing their views while preventing them from carrying on with their lives, by the same methods being used to prevent students from studying, teachers from teaching, workers from working. . . . These methods consist of intimidation, intoxication and the tyranny exerted by certain groups. For dictatorship is indeed the risk France now faces . . . I say No! The Republic will not abdicate. The people will come to their senses. Progress, independence and peace will carry the day, along with freedom. Vive la République! Vive la France!"

This remarkable strategy installs in the collective unconscious not only the fear of absence, the abstraction of this individual who steps out of the limelight for the good of the nation, "La France," but more than that, it turned de Gaulle into a living legend. He is the voice of freedom "unless there is an intention to gag the entire French people," and what a voice it is. He is the perfect embodiment of the father, the authority, the leader. De Gaulle turned the television into a medium that went beyond the image to become a verbal tool, of which the blank screen was the instrument.

Constant Vocal Characteristics

A leader's voice presents specific technical and physical characteristics. If it is to occupy the vocal space, it must have both low registers that reassure and high registers to modulate the voice. The attribution of roles in the opera illustrates this dichotomy between high and low registers. The mission of the high registers is to transmit a message. Heroes and heroines have a high tessitura; similarly in a choir, the soprano voices tell the story, while the altos establish the rhythm and envelop and support the melody. Desdemona and Othello have a high tessitura. Of course, these are but codes, and the more innovative composers break these.

Another example of this dichotomy is between bass and trebles, one that is of interest even if you're not an opera fan. In train stations, warnings against pickpockets are announced by a male voice (commuters must be reassured) while announcements about train schedules, platform numbers, or destinations are given by a female voice (commuters must be informed). The leader's voice must master navigating between these two registers; his is not a pure voice, unlike the voice of the lyrical singer. Machiavelli wrote that the prince must be both lion and fox. In other words, he must know how to roar and how to yelp. He must show his authority while reassuring the group. Besides these protective vibrations, the predator will play on fear, danger, and insecurity to consolidate his power. The politician appropriates these criteria and exploits them.

Another characteristic that is fundamental in my view is the voice of a leader must bring out the scars that life has inflicted on him, for we all have a life, and it isn't necessarily the life of a theater, cinema, or opera hero. This is a precondition for obtaining our vote. The leader's voice must be a song that resembles us. Its refrain is unique, but it carries us along, like Obama's "Yes We Can," which became the "Let It Be" of a whole generation.

Grown-Up Children

For politicians, it's a fine line that separates the voice that leads from the voice that manipulates. If leaders are to be followed, they imperatively need, beyond their personal qualities, to be in step with the living conditions of the crowd they're addressing and speak its language.

This is something that Hoover didn't understand. In 1932, in the United States, the campaign for the reelection of Herbert Hoover proved to be completely out of step with the reality of the country. Why is that? In the 1920s, Hoover's name was synonymous with prosperity. There was full employment. But then the Hoover Company laid off hordes of workers. After singing its praises, they now felt betrayed by it. Hence, at the start of the 1930s, the Hoover name, once a "lever for good," had become a dirty word, synonymous with being laid off. This analysis by Clyde Miller is very interesting, as it explains how the door was now open for Roosevelt to launch his own slogan for a new redistribution, his policy of the "New Deal," in other words, the new pact.

If leaders meet this first condition of being in step with the expectations of the masses, they may be tempted to resort to manipulation. A crowd is easily hoodwinked. Once subjugated, it behaves like an adolescent, swayed by emotion over reason and lulled by illusion, not by reality. Alchemy arises between the voice in power and the people, a phenomenon that has some parallel with the child who asks for a bedtime story and earnestly wants to believe it. When an individual is face-to-face with another, reason prevails over emotion, whereas when a leader addresses a crowd, the opposite is true.

When the words uttered by the leader touch the masses, when the leader addresses the crowd and the individual ceases to exist, that is when the leader's voice really becomes the voice of power. The individual's mechanisms of self-preservation are then almost nonexistent. The four instincts influence the masses and ignite the fire, but the voice of power is the fuse. A very strong, borderline, hypnotic charisma is required to instigate this kind of crowd reaction. Indeed, the leader's voice captivates, galvanizes, and potentiates the individual within the crowd. This energy acquires momentum and grows. The crowd turns into a mob, a monster brimming with emotion. It is "Hulk" to the tenth degree and reason ceases to exist.

The leader's very voice becomes a drug. It is a source of pleasure that triggers the release of adrenaline and dopamine. This real addiction, perverse and sneaky, feeds the crowds, who beg for more. But does one really own one's own voice? Not really, according to Montaigne: "The Word belongs as much to he who speaks it as to he who hears it." The leader's voice governs others, but it also intoxicates the leader. This was the impression Fidel Castro gave with his interminable speeches.

We're reminded of Hitler's horrible hysterical voice projecting his orgasmic vociferations—his voice was his phallus—and playing directly to the instinct of fear and to the fighting side of the instinct of self-preservation. People are often under the impression that Hitler's voice pitch was excessively high, which wasn't the case. His voice was closer to that of a tenor. With age, it dropped to baritone, as happens to most men. When he addressed the crowds, he used what is called a "head voice," talking in a voice that is louder than normal, verging on the disagreeable. With every sentence, those who listen are driven to the brink of traumatization, until, head low, they submit, tetanized, and follow the voice of their tyrant. Through his voice, Hitler deliberately sought to provoke and entertain feelings bordering on bewitchment and pain, and he is a prime example of the master manipulator.

The Codes of the Voices in Power: Is There a Casting for the Voice?

In the same way that television channels are color coded, the voices of radio channels are also coded. From the first few words uttered, we know which radio channel we're listening to. These radio voices, such as those on French radio channel for music, are the result of veritable casting auditions, comparable to the casting of Dior or Chanel models.

The voice of the man in the street and the voice of the leader have points in common, certain similarities, social rules concerning the use of certain words, and the use of the voice itself. The code of our voice is our calling card. An indicator of social background, these codes allow individuals from similar backgrounds to recognize each other. The voice creates its own codes; the power of the voice also has a cultural footprint. The voice is modified superficially like a plowed field. Culture and its geographical environment play an important role.

When we lie, the underlying psychological tension inevitably tenses our vocal cords despite us, and our voice rises. Our body language isn't "in sync" with our voice. The words say one thing; our body language says something different. This phenomenon triggers an unconscious and immediate rejection of what is said. This is seldom the case among politicians; however, they won't adopt the same manner of speech at the National Assembly, where they can modulate their voice more freely, and in a market in Saint-Malo, where sincerity is paramount; otherwise, the sanction is brutal and swift.

Our voice frequently gives away our sociocultural background, but it also reflects what we want it to say about us. Let me explain. In the exercise of our profession, our voice isn't exactly our real voice; it is the voice we choose to project, the vocal image we want others to have of us as professionals. Our authentic voice is the voice we use to talk to our self, and we alone know its real power.

An interesting observation is that the more responsibility women have in their job, the lower their voice drops. In the past 50 years, the average frequency of the female voice has dropped by three or four notes, the equivalent of around 50 Hz. Women now have warmer voices. This evolution didn't stem from a deliberate attempt to be better heard, as some have claimed on the basis that low notes carry better than high notes; it was mostly the result of a change in fashion. The shrill, high-pitched voice of the communist candidate Arlette Laguiller declaring in 1974: "I am a woman and I dare to run for the presidency of this republic of men" would fall very flat in 2017.

First and foremost, one must know how to control one's voice. Remember Ségolène Royal's retort: "I'm not angry, Mr. Sarkozy." The second she said that, she had lost out.

Controlling one's voice can be learned. The higher the pitch, with a strong intensity, the more unpleasant and irritating it is; the lower the pitch, the softer the voice, and the lower the volume, the more reassuring it is. It doesn't batter the eardrums; it is in harmony with a pleasant listening experience. The voice is frequency, strength, harmony, rhythm, and silence.

Leaders may use different vocal codes; they don't address the media and their supporters in the same tone. To communicate well with a group, it is crucial to know what the code of that group is, be it a group of lawyers, doctors, politicians, or rap artists.

Léon Schwarzenberg, an eminent oncologist I knew well when I was a young assistant at Villejuif, lasted a mere fortnight as Minister of Health. He lacked the vocal code of the politician, the voice of diplomacy; his was the code of truthful medicine. He was in favor of straight-talk, of authentic communication. His message was intended more for the ears of the sick than for the ears of politicians or a political party. Admittedly, his code, the code of a scientist and humanist, despite its rules, also had its limits.

On another register, Bernard Tapie, an important businessman (ADIDAS), became the Minister for Urban Affairs but also only lasted a few months in that privileged circle of ministers. He had the code that favored straight-talk, with the vocal footprint of the street urchin. The social code of his voice was too obvious to be widely accepted: "a street code."

These examples of very different personalities illustrate that the code of the spoken voice requires knowledge, in its broadest sense, of the person or persons addressed. If I know the code, I can identify with the group and the group can identify with me. I'm safe, and the image I project of the leader is protected. Today more than ever, the voice, not the clothes, makes the man. The voice becomes clannish; it refers back to a dominant group. Silvio Berlusconi was as arrogant as Bernard Tapie, and these two men exploited the media remarkably with today's weapons; moreover, as a journalist wrote in the magazine *Le Point* in 1994, "Both men are explorers, recycling for the cathodic tube and the elections the misgivings of the collective unconscious in a period of crisis." But Berlusconi for his part knew the political code; he was an insider, one of them.

The politician's voice must be received across a very wide range. It needs to be understood by all, whatever the social status, education, or intellect at the receiving end.

But the voice also answers to some universal codes. Listen to Charlie Chaplin in *The Dictator*, mimicking Hitler addressing the masses! Not a word of German is spoken, there is no language, no syntax, no identifiable meaning. Just music and prosody. One can hear the pseudo-words, the silences, the breaks, the vociferations that say it all. The code of the dictator's voice is clearly recognizable.

The power of the voice highlights, sometimes outrageously, words that are set off by the tone of voice. Words have an undeniable role to play in communication or as an instrument of our thinking. One of the main roles of the voice is to transmit words, and it also multiplies their strength and their impact. Indeed, a single word has both a form and a meaning, a signifier and a signified; the same word can be interpreted in different ways. Its meaning can vary according to who utters it. Sometimes it is ambiguous and causes a misunderstanding. This faculty of the voice to offer several commentaries and elucidations is a permanent source of creativity for man. Words are defined by other words. They're only put to use within this closed system. The word is kneaded, shaken, and molded by the musicality of the voice; it influences, persuades or misleads, commands or entraps. The voice, composed of words and their capacity to express thoughts, forces its power on the other person, on a collective, but also on oneself.

Fashion and the Voices in Power

"Lay to rrrrrrrrrest here, Jean Moulin, with your terrrrrible procession." The words are strung out, giving resonance to every breath of the icy wind in this temple of great men. The "R" rumbles like a drum roll, all the "A"s seemingly circumflexed: "Here we have the funeral march of the ashes . . . those of Victor Hugo and *Les Misérables*, those of Jaurès, over whom Justice keeps vigil, may they rest with their long procession of disfigured shadows." The day is December 19, 1964. André Malraux pronounces his famous discourse on the occasion of the presentation of Jean Moulin's ashes at the Pantheon, his famous voice theatrical, almost wavering, like the flame of remembrance. Using the familiar "tu" form to address the deceased, that day it was he who passed into history. His voice marked a whole period of history. Indeed, Sarah Bernhardt's recordings and Malraux's nasal, quavering inflections show only very minor differences.

A quarter of a century later, on November 9, 1988, it is Jean Monnet's turn to enter the Pantheon. In the bluish halo of the EU flags, François Mitterrand addresses his fellow citizens, the Europeans. This time, he keeps the wording simple, his voice devoid of emphasis: "Each one here symbolizes a moment in History, an attitude toward life, a way of being: Jean Moulin and the French Resistance for the love of the nation, René Cassin, to defend and improve the Law, Jean Monnet, Europe and the construction of peace." History has become modest. May 1968 has left its stamp. The world changes, and so does the way the voice is used.

Just as a man's voice evolves over the years, the voice itself has a history, made of disruptions and continuities. From the frescoes at Lascaux to Rembrandt's portraits, including Michelangelo's sculptures, calligraphy, or printing, man has never ceased to inscribe his memory, but prior to the 20th century, there is no trace of the voice in our collective heritage. From hence on, great voices can be listened to and transmitted to future generations, on an equal footing with all other human activities.

We discovered how to trap the voice. When we listen to a famous voice that has passed on; we resurrect it. The past becomes a present image, more exactly; these present vibrations solicit our memory. Hearing someone's voice is more instructive than looking at a photograph; the person seems to spring back to life, to be with us.

Malraux's voice is theatrical, well projected, the voice of a talented comedian who could do without a microphone. The politicians from that era all sound as if they are straight out of the Cours Simon, the famed Parisian drama school created in 1925. Some of these voices have a bantering tone, like Jean Gabin when he says, "T'as de beaux yeux, tu sais" ("You have beautiful eyes, you know"), or pronounce their Rs from the back of the throat, like Raimu; others emphasize double letters, like Pierre Fresnay in *La Grande Illusion*, or Louis Jouvet in *Knock*, with his famous "Ça vous grrratouille ou ça vous chatouille?" ("Does it scrrratch you or does it tickle?"). These voices are all typical of their time, which they represent far better than any photograph or image from a film. The very first vibrations of these actors' voices awaken memories for us. Their physiognomy, their gestures, and their diction are suited to being received from afar. In their day, a microphone was an accessory that was still rarely used, and then only to modify the strength and power of the voice rather than its timbre.

Back then, the men giving speeches, men I would almost describe as preachers, were orators. They had to project their voice beyond imaginary footlights, and in the absence of decor and lighting, this was probably harder to do than in any theater. In fact, the barer the setting, the more eloquent they needed to be, verging on caricature. The best voices take on multiple characters, such as de Gaulle's voice, at times the victorious general full of panache, at other times the honest family man in a three-piece suit giving reassurance in a paternal tone. When the ashes of Jean Moulin were laid to rest, the general, dignified and imperturbable, appeared in uniform, practically for the last time. André Malraux's features show the scars of past battles, while the solemnity of the present moment weighs heavy on his shoulders. His face solemn, his jaw tense, he speaks of fighting for a better future in the name of the past. Bright-eyed, he holds forth, however, in the style of a Comédie Française comedian, his sepia-colored words worthy of the French Academy.

Less than four years later, this same square before the Pantheon is invaded by chanting students brandishing cobblestones: "Ten years is enough!" Theirs is the voice of a new world, young and swift that has made more progress in a decade than in the past century. A new vocal timbre, a new rhythm are heard. The specter of war has vanished, and the feeding instinct, though not completely gone, has diminished considerably. What stands out is a new energy; enjoy life is the new mantra, and fear of scarcity has practically disappeared. The West puts a premium on appearance; a healthy and athletic appearance increasingly finds favor, along with bodybuilding. In the 1970s, a new trend, already well established in the United States, emerges in France—people are more self-aware, cultivate their image, and manage their voice.

At the start of the 20th century, Max Weber, one of the founding fathers of sociology, gave a definition of the power of those who govern that is still apt today. According to him, the legitimacy of those who rule has its roots in three types of legitimacy: traditional authority, rational authority, and charismatic or seductive authority. The media have only amplified the importance of this phenomenon. The same message can be repeated throughout the day. You can listen to it in the car, on television, or on a smartphone. On one hand, the crowd loses something of its essence as a physical collectivity and becomes a virtual one; on the other, it continues to behave like a crowd due to the considerable impact of the audiovisual media. The individual knows he is one among many auditors, and that feeling of belonging to a wider group confers upon him power-by-proxy. The interview method has been marking time since the 1980s. The political duel is now envisaged as a gladiator fight, and television viewers expect demise.

The weight of media criticism is continually increasing, its lens now encompassing one's physical appearance and, especially, one's voice and body language. From the 1980s onward, the voice of those in power is no longer theatrical, as in films; it is shown with greater intimacy, as in an American full-screen shot: The politician can be seen and heard up close, maybe with his supporters. After 2000, I would say we're approaching hand-to-hand combat, especially as regards Nicholas Sarkozy. Whether with a journalist or with a political rival, a fight is never off the cards with him, and the television viewer loves a good verbal joust.

Leaders have taken up sports activities, are careful about their figure, and make public their way of life, and by the same token, their voice has also changed. It has evolved from a theatrical, conversational style to a simple conversational style; the imaginary setting of their discourse is no longer a stage, but a television studio or a radio station, with a small audience on set. Hence, the new importance of a good microphone and a talented sound engineer is obvious to transmit "the voice." The microphone commonly favored is a Shure SM57. Manufactured by Shure, it is dynamic, unidirectional, and conceived for recording both vocal and instrumental sounds. It has been the official microphone of the U.S. president since 1965; all public addresses made by American presidents since then have been recorded with this microphone. It renders the full frequency range of the voice. It allows one to isolate the main source of sound, while muting any background noise. It reduces parasite manipulation noises thanks to a pneumatic antishock system. The message being transmitted must at all cost be pleasant to listen to acoustically. Technological progress does not only accompany social change, but it is also a determining factor in this change. People have born witness to the fact that at the start of Hitler's political career, when he spoke in cafés, his voice was very simple. His orator voice only emerged once he started addressing thousands of people. Without technical support, the voice only carries 30 to 50 meters, hence the need for a microphone.

But the first microphones didn't immediately produce any changes. They amplified the sound but distorted the voice; lacking balance, the voice lost sincerity. Consequently, it was better to do without and work one's voice as on a stage. I recall my venerable teachers at the medical school I attended at Rue des Saints-Pères, obstinately refusing to consider using a microphone for their lectures, while the younger generation couldn't do without it.

Microphones and loudspeaker advances changed everything, once not just the Beatles, Ray Charles, or the Rolling Stones, but also leaders, were able to use them without losing any of their singularity—in all its senses—and communicated their emotion to their audience. The best example I know of remains Kennedy's speech in Berlin, in June 1963, when the president exclaimed, "Ich bin in Berliner" to the assembled crowd, instead of "Ich bin *ein* Berliner." Never mind that Goethe's language had just been violated; everyone applauded, and so ensured Kennedy's triumph.

His voice was low-key, conversational; he was an American in Germany making the effort to speak the local "lingo." The microphone saved him. Indeed, without a microphone, in theatrical mode, he would have been booed; I'm convinced of that, just like the stage actor who makes a mess of his lines or the opera singer who hits a false note.

The microphone ushered familiarity onto the political scene, a proximity that lends softness to the sound rendering, like a troubadour rocking us with his pianissimo. Like the crooner, the politician shares his plan for reform in a confidential tone. Kennedy was the Sinatra of the political world. When he addressed a crowd, he was talking to every person there. He brought intimacy into the collective arena.

But this intimacy that has crept into the relationship between politicians and their auditors (or television viewers) in this virtual crowd has a terrible downside. In my view, if today the private life of leaders is so exposed, it is also because of the changes that technical advances have brought about in the voice and that have brought politicians closer to us. It is no longer the voice of France addressing the French; it is the voice of an individual talking to us, with his failings, his faults, and his qualities. Although leaders' voices have become more approachable, more familiar, they still stand out because of their vocal charisma. Speech after speech, the politician has come off his pedestal; when de Gaulle said "La France," he was France, and little was known about him. Nicholas Sarkozy addresses himself to "the French," his fellow men, divorcees who feel good because they have time to go jogging on Sundays and don't smoke. As for President Hollande, he uses a simple vocabulary that everyone can understand, with no emphasis, and he can contradict himself like any Tom, Dick, and Harry. He probably is "a normal president," as he claims, but normal as against what and whom?

May 1968 instigated social changes, but it was only smoothing the way for what, for me, was the real revolution: the opening up of the sound space for the H. F. radio channel, by François Mitterrand, in 1981. Until then, auditors had to make do with the medium wave transmissions diffused by ORTF (Office de

Radiodiffusion-Télévision Française). Medium wave can't carry all sound pulses; it transmits only certain registers of frequencies. If the voice were a spectrum of colors, in medium wave, the orator would be color blind vocally. Thanks to FM's ability to modulate frequency, in FM the purity of the voice is transmitted with near perfect integrity.

When Mitterrand pays homage to Jean Monnet, his voice doesn't seek to impose; it no longer needs to. The injunctions and lyrical flights personified by Malraux have been replaced by facts and symbols. Here, too, the keyword is proximity. When I listen without interruption to François Hollande while driving, as on a misty morning in October 2014, I listen with half an ear. Our leaders no longer expect us to hang on their every word. They themselves are used to speaking incessantly, not vacuously, but to occupy the media space. This space is saturated with the voices of politicians, be it the president or his ministers, the opposition or trade unionists, at the expense of artists and culture. But how can politicians be heard, when on certain radio and television channels, their voices are just background noise punctuated by advertisements? Such is the problem our male and female politicians currently face. There is only one remedy: to repeat as often as possible a message that is as simple as possible, a bit like a bass line in a melody. Leaders constantly comment on specific problems and events, but what really matters is the refrain they strike up at every turn. In 1995, it was "the social fracture"; in 2007, "work harder, earn more"; or in 2008, Obama's "Yes We Can." Welcome to the era of relentless repetition, of repetitiousness on a global scale. You'll notice that these refrains are increasingly sterile, not because of any shortage of ideas or because of faulty syntax, but because the greater the flow of information, the harder it is for us to recall it. There's no point in bemoaning this, but neither does it pass unnoticed. While the spoken word and speeches proliferate, catchphrases and watchwords are repeated again and again, like an advertising jingle. No need to read into this an attempt to manipulate or to influence through subliminal messages, nor should one see the devil's work in everything related to the media; it's simply *Homo politicus* adapting to his environment, to his history that varies from one country to another. For all the popularity of Obama's "Yes We Can," its equivalent would never have worked in France. Obama speaks like a preacher, in a voice that is often monochord, the tonality spiritual and moralizing, addressing himself directly to the American people, leaving them room to dream and to envisage the future. In France, homeland of secularism, this kind of politician has yet to emerge.

Neither is it possible to turn the clock back. Today, Mitterrand possibly wouldn't even get past the primary elections. His speeches are too long. These days, long speeches are the hallmark of poor content. Similarly, politicians with a theatrical elocution criticized for speaking too loudly also don't go down well. Big political rallies are getting rare. They mainly serve to show the good health of the speaker and his faculty for speaking at length without getting out of breath. If supporters were already convinced, now they leave reassured.

The political voice is undoubtedly subject to fashion trends. "Fashion" may be a futile term; nevertheless, it is pertinent. If politicians, male or female, want to succeed, they must keep up with the times and be familiar with their environment and the sound space they evolve in. No one expects them to be a rap artist, but they must understand the rap artist and speak a language he can understand. The theatricals of earlier politicians, the Gabins and the Jouvets of the political scene, have been replaced by serial actors. We see them day in day out, for no apparent reason. They will never be heroes. Among the voices in power, if politicians or leaders are to win, they need to elicit a certain admiration, a certain respect, and be liked. Through their voice, they convey their thinking and, especially, their emotion. The very true example is Emmanuel Macron, president of France at the age of 39. His voice is sincere and true, and he is an expert, a man from the people, a man who gives dreams to the young generation. This young generation lives in an open world from digital technology, but they don't forget their roots.

CHAPTER 3

The Essential Is Invisible

The voice is the body's intangible and omnipresent musical instrument, its alchemy born from an alliance of body and soul. The voice is immanence through its emotion and transcendence through the metamorphosis of the body's breath of life into vibrations.

There are as many different voices as there are grains of sand in the ocean. We are seven billion *Homo vocalis*, each with our own distinct voice, our own vibrations. The voice transduces ecstasy in prayer or in incantation, also in hope or in sacrifice in certain rituals, such as voodoo. The vibrations of *Homo vocalis* are an inconstant balance between silence and sound, inspiration and expiration, yin and yang. Thus, the voice is a message that connects man with himself and with others.

Of our various means of communication, the voice is the most intimate and the most naked manifestation of our essential self. It is in us; it reveals our highest spiritual conscience. It allows us to dialogue with our inner self and also to express our every emotion, our every feeling. The mystery of the voice is part of the mystery of life, a sort of emotional hologram.

Of Gods and Voices

In antiquity, the voice inspired in man the most phantasmagorical stories. All the mythologies narrate them. In our part of the world, the great founding fictions are called *The Iliad* and *The Odyssey*, *The Enid*, *The Metamorphoses*, and so on.

Witness Orpheus seducing the gods with his voice to obtain their clemency. His singing could charm wild animals, the trees and the stones, even the guardians of the Underworld, who, after hearing him sing, agree to set free the beautiful Eurydice. The mermaids try to attract Ulysses, who is so charmed by their bewitching chant that he has to ask his crew to tie him to the mast in order not to succumb to it. Inspired by the Muses, Echo, a nymph of the woods and springs, is able through her endless chatter to distract Hera's attention from the frolicking of her husband, Zeus, with beautiful mortals. When the goddess discovers the subterfuge, in a rage she punishes Echo by depriving her of her own voice. Hera passed sentence on her with these words: "You will always have the last word, but no power to speak first." It was condemning her to relentlessly echo the voice of others. Echo is to the voice what Narcissus is to the image, but he disappeared, whereas the personified echo still roams the mountains. Hold on to the symbolism of the message here. Images are fleeting, whereas vibrations leave their footprint in space.

Zeus, another figure from Greek mythology, is the master of all voices. His spoken word has public authority; it is *muthos*, "the voice to which public speech belongs."

Zeus asks Hephaestus to knead water and clay to create Pandora, the first woman. The gods have breathed her human voice into her; she is goddess of the Earth and presides over fertility.

Sybil, Apollo's priestess, allows mortals to communicate with the gods through her voice. She is the detainer of certain secrets. She delivers messages to the gods through trances, songs, and dances. Already of a certain age, this prophetess or echo of the oracles is an instrument of revelation considered to be an emanation of divine wisdom. She talks in the first person and acknowledges the originality of her prophecy and the independent nature of her answers, which at times can be really "wacky" and require serious decoding. Her enigmatic language is open to numerous interpretations. An oft-quoted example is this prophecy, addressed to a soldier: "*Ibis redibis non morieris in bello.*" If a pause is made before "non," the sentence means: "You will go, you will return, you will not die in battle." But if the pause comes after "non," the sentence means: "You will go, you will not return, you will die in battle." This goes to show how very important the vocal melody is!

The role of the Pythia was different. Hers was an institutional status associated with the Delphi sanctuary. She is only a spokeswoman for the gods, answering questions posed to her.

Diodorus of Sicily writes that near Delphi, vapor gushed out of the earth, sowing confusion in people's mind and disturbing their senses. A shepherd guarding his herd of goats nearby noticed that when his goats approached these vapors, they would leap in the air and become frenetic, all the while bleating strangely. He himself then ingested some vapor and also began to jump about, in the grip of an unusual euphoria. He experienced visions, spoke gibberish, and came to the conclusion that something divine had invested this fissure. News of this soon spread across Greece. People saw in these strange events the hands of the gods. A few reckless souls rushed there to breathe in the vapors. They fell into the fissure and perished. It was then decided that a woman would become the priestess of this place, the Pythia of Delphi. Only she would be entitled to serve as the oracle, acting as a go-between for people wanting to question Apollo. A tripod is made for her to sit on and placed above the vent. Seated on the tripod, which has been perforated, she is swathed in these vapors, which some people believe must rise through her back passage and her sexual organs in order to be fully effective. The woman becomes a prophet. Her voice changes. The timbre is different. She goes into trance. Most impressive is the fact that her lips don't move when she speaks. Her voice seems to come from elsewhere. It must be the gods speaking through her! Could the Pythia be the ventriloquist with the most closely guarded secret in history? The mystery of these voices was only pierced centuries later, something I shall go into later on.

If the Sybil played the role of a spokeswoman interceding between the gods and mortals, has this role not been replicated under different skies, in the voodoo rituals of Benin, Haiti, and Brazil? Do these incantations not seek to make the gods speak out, give new life to the elders, and, through their chanting, incarnate the manifestation and presence of the gods?

Among the Dogon: Voice Is God

The voice is sovereign in Dogon mythology. It has absolute power. This tribe lives on the arid plateau of Bandiagara, in Mali. The Dogon people have constructed a cosmogony so fantastic it seems straight out of a science fiction novel. At the core of their philosophy is the voice, both sacred element and creator. This philosophy is completed by two principles. The principle of the necessary duality and complementarity of beings and of things, and the principle of a vital energy that animates all elements created, from minerals to man.

The god of the Dogon rules over the spoken word. He fashions the original placenta. The spoken word is the symbol of fertility. An empty word doesn't allow others to create or to procreate. A rich, sincere word impregnates the placenta and offers it to Din, the chosen man among men. He and he alone can develop the human voice. Without voice, man doesn't exist! For Din, the power of the voice depends on water, giver of life. If one is dehydrated, one cannot speak. Water lends the voice fluidity and assurance and allows it to impose itself. The rhythm of the voice is like a river, like a torrent, like the tide. If the water isn't pure, the voice is insincere; it is false, deceitful, and opaque. Fire is the source that imparts the voice with emotion. The spoken word can be warm, cordial, brutal, or cold. The earth gives the voice substance, shaping the scaffolding of man's being. The air is the ultimate source of the spoken word and bestows charm upon it. This philosophy of the Dogon, a people in complete symbiosis with nature, in harmony with the constellations, and especially with Sirius, the brightest star of all, is remarkable; it reveals the extent to which the transmission of knowledge and experience is tightly interwoven with this vibrational "DNA" that is the voice.

The Dogon reproduce not only the human voice but also the breeze, noises made by animals, and they translate—though "exorcise" is a more apt description—man's anguish, claiming to be man's messengers. They aren't the creators of the words, chants, cries, and onomatopoeia they pronounce; they're a relay for these incantations. The power of their voice becomes absolute ("It isn't me, it's the elder"); they're inhabited by a voice.

Here, the notion of transmitter and receiver becomes fundamental. The transmitter is commonly the person creating the voice. That may be an actor, but an actor takes on a role (for example, that of a hypnotizer) and is identified with it. The Dogon witchdoctor is both transmitter and receiver. He is a relay station—a simile would be a postman opening your mail to read it to you. Thus, is anguish exorcised? Here, the individual is at the service of the individual in contrast to other instances, in which the individual feeds on the collective.

Diphonic Chanting

The diphonic chants of the Tibetan monks have long been an enigma for laryngologists such as I. This unique voice, which could almost be from another planet, with a sacred resonance, was a startling discovery for me when I had occasion to examine a master of this art, Trân Quang Hai. One morning in February 1987, Trân Quang Hai phoned me and came to my surgery, accompanied by his wife, Bach Yên. I examined him. He presents presented the symptoms of a banal pharyngitis. With his agreement, we explored his larynx using nasal video endoscopy. A wonderful opportunity for me to see up close the mystery of the diphonic voice and understand how this intonation is produced!

I introduce the fiberscope into his right nasal fossa. The video enabled me to follow on screen the progress of the fiberscope. Once at the top of the nasopharynx, the roof of the pharynx, the fiberscope continued its progression behind the uvula before reaching the larynx. I then asked him to sing "Ode to Joy" in a normal voice. The soft palate, the tongue, and the pharynx all behaved normally. The vocal cords came together, closing off the larynx thanks to those tiny joints, the arytenoids, and began to vibrate. The muscle bundles above, known as the false vocal cords, didn't contract, which is normal. Trân Quang Hai then sang "Ode to Joy" in a diphonic voice.

What happened next was amazing. The vocal cords contracted very tightly, as did the false vocal cords. The arytenoids came together, as usual when sound is emitted, but now they tipped slightly forward, almost masking the vocal cord. I found myself obliged to lower the fiberscope to a point three to four mm above the arytenoids. Here I was able to trap the musical instrument of the larynx. What was vibrating was extraordinary. Later, in 2007, filming at four thousand images per second, I saw that, contrary to expectation, the ventricular bands, the vocal cords, and the mucous membrane of the arytenoids all vibrated. The whole larynx became an instrument that vibrated all over!

Examining Trân, I also noticed in his athlete's pharynx the same structures and torsions of the tongue, or of the soft palate, as can be observed in ventriloquists. Like a Sherlock Holmes, I had discovered the mystery of the diphonic voice. I observed closely this impressive technique at work, its laryngeal biomechanics so complex and intriguing.

This singing is variably called diphonic, biformantic, or diplophonic. The common denominator is the position of the tongue in relation to the larynx and to the pharynx, which allows the singer to maintain the bumblebee, a buzzing sound in a very low frequency, while producing the melody. The bumblebee is the first fundamental tone. In a sense, one could say it provides the basic structure for the second tone. Maintaining the bumblebee sound at a constant pitch, in the same frequency, with the same volume, on a single exhale, enables the melody to develop above it. This technique, which has long been in the service of Buddhist philosophy, aspires to be the instrument of immanence, whereas our European civilization is more oriented toward transcendence.

In the Hindu religion, the voice is also a fundamental element. In Sanskrit, the syllable "aum" represents the divine primitive vibration, and when pronounced in 40 different ways, it becomes a source of energy. Here, the voice has power both in its immanence and in its transcendence.

These diphonic chants have an unusual power. Not just through the message they carry, but also because of the technique they require. The Tibetan monks aren't alone in practicing this vocal oddity; it can also be found among certain Mongols, notably the Tuvas. The technique used in diphonic singing bears similarities with the technique used by ventriloquists. The 3D images I'm now scanning are practically the same as the ones produced by that magician of the voice, the ventriloquist. The resonance chambers are similar in both cases.

A God and Voices

Invisible, intangible, and immaterial, by its very nature the voice opens the doors of the sacred. Our very first experience of the voice is also steeped in mystery. Well before all mystics, is the fetus not the first to hear voices, in the mother's womb?

Ethereal, the voice rises naturally toward the heavens, and in the three monotheist religions, it also descends from the heavens to bring the Word of God unto men. From the archangel Gabriel to the Books of Revelation, nowhere in the Bible is a reference to a voice challenged, be it the Word of God, often described as "powerful" or "calm," the voice of the patriarchs, of King Solomon or of Saint John. When the Jews in Jerusalem sent priests and Levites to ask Saint John, "Who are you?" he answered, "I am the voice of He who shouts in the desert." In the Bible, the divine word is often put forward to validate mystery. God spoke, "Let there be Light" and from his Word "There was light." Do the Ten Commandments not mean "the Ten Words" in Aramaic? Since the earliest times, religious canticles have been punctuated with *Alleluias*, vowels combining to lend support to man's voice. The voice dresses up with words, but as in other domains, the musicality of the discourse takes precedence over the sense of the words. Religion can't exist without words, but the opposite also holds true. Synagogue, church, cathedral, mosque, temple—so many different architectures, all of them envisioned capturing the voice of the faithful and making it resonate.

The Church has always been suspicious of the voice, as indeed of words and song. Why is that? Because the voice can bring joy, as it can suffering or distress, its purity is doubted; yet God can't be praised without it. To escape this contradiction, voices were classified according to their degree of purity.

In this context, Jews, Christians, and Muslims concur, each in their own way, that men must be warned against the seductive dangers of the female voice. A woman's voice is judged to be intrinsically erotic and troubling. She can therefore not be authorized to call the faithful to prayer or to lead religious services. For in the religious context, the power of the voice is exercised principally in prayer or in the recital of sacred texts (when the voice is used on other occasions in a religious context, for instance, to preach or to deliver a homily or a sermon, the same rules apply as in any other public speaking).

In Judaism, the Hazzan (the cantor) reads the Torah, or rather sings the Torah, in accordance with strictly defined musical codes. Indeed, the Jewish liturgy is for the most part sung or recited in rhythm with traditional melodies. In Islam, the muezzin is the person appointed at the mosque to call Muslims to prayer at least five times a day, often from the top one of the mosque's minarets, the muezzin appeals. He is chosen for his voice and good character.

In the quest for pure voices, the Christian culture stands alone in having showcased the singing voice of children, considered to be the perfect instrument to embody the angelic ideal of the Christian ritual.

In the Protestant churches, the power of the voice is professed loud and clear. For Calvin, "a man's voice is far more excellent than any musical instrument, for these are dead things." The faithful therefore sing *a capella*, for praising God and praying to God should not be done through music, whether it is delegated to a musician or to a cantor.

The same is true of the Orthodox Church, where the banishment of all musical instruments has favored the development of an extraordinary polyphony. The chanting of sacred texts in orthodox music is therefore a purely vocal art. The human voice is used very differently in the Church and in profane matters. The voice is transfigured by the tone and becomes the instrument through which man expresses his praise to his creator. Sacred chanting is born from an interaction of voices that enables each individual to resonate collectively.

Since millennia, sacred music and sacred chants have reached the highest levels of art. They gave rise to the opera, which in turn has been able to embody the power of the voice through its capacity to take it to ethereal heights, overcoming Earth's gravity.

Hypnotic Power

Hypnosis is still today often associated with magical powers, yet it is a natural phenomenon, and one increasingly used in the medical field. A hypnotic state is simply a modified state of conscience. Quite distinct from sleep, it is a state that we experience several times a day, to different degrees, every time our mind is "elsewhere."

A little history: The term "hypnosis" was invented in 1843 by the Scottish doctor James Braid, worthy heir to Mesmer, who made us rediscover the practical application of hypnosis, on the border between science and ShowTime.

France has played a fundamental role in the development of hypnosis in the psychiatric field, both at the Pitié-Salpêtrière Hospital in Paris and at the Nancy School of Psychiatry. Today, hypnosis is used in psychiatry and for anesthesia. MRI techniques have enhanced our understanding of it. Under hypnosis, specific areas of the brain are activated, different from those activated when we relax or sleep.

In the normal waking state, there are two types of conscience. The first is "critical." It looks at details, analyses, dissects, observes, and protects us. This state of conscience is colder and more distant than the second one, which one could call "hypnotic"; this one focuses on the whole picture, is more dream-like, and feeds on creativity and imagination. It is "warmer" and more natural. During the course of a day, we fluctuate between these two states. We do so naturally, to different degrees, and more or less adequately. It is this second state of hypnotic conscience that is provoked for a specific purpose.

The basic principles of this "hypnotic" conscience are dissociation and sensoriality. The term "dissociation" describes the feeling that "my body is here, but my mind is elsewhere."

The hypnotic phenomenon is accompanied by an altered state of conscience and memory. It allows a keener sensitivity to suggestion and to visualization. You find yourself plunged in a world in which the answers to questions may seem strange, bizarre, and unsuspected, and ideas may seem unfamiliar and even incongruous.

In my surgery, it was my anesthetist, Bernard, who made me discover how the hypnotic state facilitates anesthesia and also lightens and often modifies the patient's perception of pain.

The first time I saw Bernard hypnotize a patient before anesthesia, I was taken by surprise, as no one had forewarned me. Bernard asked us all to be quiet. I thought there might be a problem with the anesthesia, but he explained he was going to induce a light trance in the patient to relax her. For his voice to be effective, he must talk to her in a low, gentle tone and make her state of mind receptive. The key to this is to talk to her in rhythm with her breathing, more specifically, on her exhale. Indeed, a deep exhale is an indispensable element for relaxation. She can then relax and focus fully on his words. There are no parasite noises. The mind settles.

A very important element is taking into consideration the state of the patient. Repeating "Calm down, relax, all is well" in a soothing voice to a patient who is stressed out and agitated won't get the desired result; it can even have a negative effect. For all that there is a trance state in which everything positive and pleasant is enhanced, there is also a trance state in which all negative elements are amplified. In such a case, one has to take the patient's state into account by meeting the patient halfway, adopting a rather energetic tone and a faster rate of speech. Once the patient and the therapist are on the same wavelength, the therapist can progressively diminish the rhythm and intensity of his voice to bring the patient into a more appeased state. To do this, *pacing* is used, a breathing technique in which the therapist synchronizes his breathing with the patient's breathing. Even if the therapist doesn't speak, the simple fact of pacing is very appeasing for the patient, especially in the case of a difficult patient in the grip of severe stress.

An example is appropriate here to better illustrate these states of conscience. When I'm driving alone in my car on the highway and I'm bored, I can let my mind drift without falling asleep. If I need to overtake, I can easily "reassociate" myself; I put on my indicator, overtake, and get back into the slow lane. Once conditions are quiet again, I can "wander off" again in my mind.

In the context of hypnotic trance, the anesthetist uses a tone that is persuasive without being coercive to ask the patient to focus on a pleasant memory, using only his or her senses: "You're not going to think about it, you're going to *relive* it through your senses."

During a hypnosis session, the power of the voice is remarkable in that its usage seems contrary to expectation.

In everyday life, the voice uses affect to emphasize its power, yet for hypnosis to be effective, the voice must be totally neutral, betraying no emotion, monotone, monochord, and monochrome. The voice of the therapist seems disembodied; it needs to leave the center stage to the patient's emotions. Nothing must be imposed on the patient. The voice accompanies the exhale; thus its action coincides with the patient letting go and appeals directly to nonemotional internal resonances. One can hypothesize that the monochord timbre and tone of the hypnotist's voice pierces the conscious mind of the person being hypnotized without making it "disappear."

Another point: In order to avoid the slightest upset that might disturb the hypnotic process, words must always be used in their positive sense. For example, if you say to a patient, "Don't worry, this won't hurt, it won't be long," the message retained will be "worry," "hurt," and "long." Bear in mind that the patient is likely to be in a negative trance state and therefore more receptive to these "suggestions" of worry and pain than when in a more neutral state. The choice of words is, however, less important than the tone used. It's the lulling tone that will really accompany this pleasant little escapade, giving the feeling that one is protected by this "voice" that guides and reassures.

People with a modicum of experience can also practice self-hypnosis. In that case, patient and therapist are but one.

Due to their monochord characteristic, Gregorian or Tibetan chants can produce the right conditions for another form of hypnosis. Listening to them can lead to an ecstatic state. More generally speaking, it seems to me that this is the effect all music lovers are after, as music plunges one into a peculiar state that can go as far as a trance. This underscores the accessibility of hypnosis to all and sundry.

CHAPTER 4

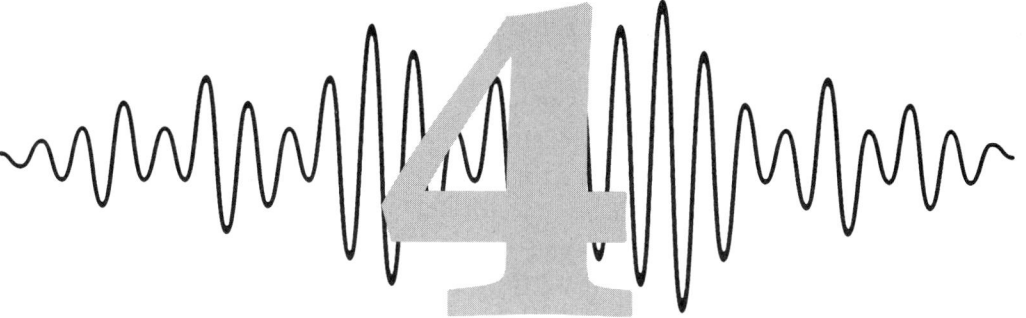

The Voice Must Go On

In the beginning is the voice. It is through the voice's very first cry that we manifest life.

If the voice is our first means of communication, it is also through the voice that we belong to the world. Since time immemorial, men have sought to imitate nature and its acoustic environment; vocal traditions have sprung up for this purpose, generating a wealth of songs and vocal games. All civilizations, from the most primitive to the most sophisticated, bear witness to this. Man adds his voice to the song of the world, as if to tame it.

The voice accompanies all our existential rituals. It is also one of the forms of expression that is most equally shared between the two sexes. Women feature as prominently in the practice of the vocal arts as do men. Even when relegated to the domestic front, this art is a factor of equality in societies that don't always practice gender equality.

Aside from singing for oneself or in a group—lullabies, ritualistic chants, or songs for specific occasions—the voice is also a profession. Reserved to a select few, the profession imposes constant practice, a solid training, working to deadlines, the risk of sanctions—in other words, all the prerequisites of any art form in which emotion is both a means and the objective. It isn't for private consumption; it is intended for the ears of a public who will pass judgment on it. The singing or spoken voice is an art only because it is subject to and subjected to interpretation, in all the senses of the word. It is above all a technique, one that requires tenacious application, willpower, and passion. The ventriloquist, the imitator, the actor, or the singer must ensure their voice is heard and resonates if it is to reveal the full extent of its power. Thus, the interpreter is condemned to surpass himself and to push back the human limits of the voice, as singing is undoubtedly the most accomplished and the most fascinating of the voice's manifestations.

The Ventriloquist

The United States has incredible talents as these two very famous ventriloquists Valentine Vox in the late 90s or Dunham now with his famous puppet, a skull. In France, one of them is represented by Marc Métral. In 2014, this illusionist in his 60s drew attention on British television by seducing the public and the jury on *Britain's Got Talent*. He is the first ventriloquist to use a live animal, a little dog, in a show. A familiar face in cabarets and circuses the world over, this wasn't his coming out; he had already performed in front of Lady Diana in 1988 and also at the Olympia and the Moulin Rouge. Nowadays, Christian Gabriel is one of the best with his puppet, a monkey named Freddy, and I did most of my research with him. A young guy came on the field: Jeff Panacloc who is incredible.

The ventriloquist's art still fascinates the crowds as much as ever, even though the mystery it was shrouded in for centuries has long been pierced. Indeed, this magician of the voice, this modern entertainer, was considered before as a sorcerer invested with a supernatural vocal power over men. As touched upon earlier in relation to the prophetesses of antiquity, ventriloquists represented occult forces; they communicated with the dead, making them talk and predicting the future.

The engastrimyth, or ventriloquist, is considered the equivalent of a god. But thanks to his oracles, the ventriloquist may also freely express the people's grievances and may sometimes take a stand against the political powers that be, since it isn't really the ventriloquist talking. His role is first and foremost spiritual. The origin of the word is crystal clear: from the Greek *egastrimitos* —*gaster* (stomach) and *mythos* (voice). Hippocrates tried his hand at describing it. The ventriloquist has a voice that comes from the stomach; it is the voice of the soul emitted by an internal force. Hippocrates simply picked up on an evocation in the Bible (Isaiah 29:4): "Brought low, you will speak from the ground; your speech will mumble out of the dust. Your voice will come ghostlike from the earth; out of the dust your speech will whisper."

Still from the Bible, in the Book of Samuel, a ventriloquist makes an appearance in the episode concerning Saul, who comes to consult the magician Endor, in her day the most famous necromancer and reputed to have the "ôbh," "the gift of divination by evoking the dead." King Saul, abandoned by God, attempts to communicate with the defunct prophet Samuel, seeking a message from him. Samuel had ordained him king when Saul was 40. A voice from elsewhere answers: "Your army will be beaten by the Philistines. You will lose your sceptre." The necromancer is stone-faced; her lips don't move. Whence does the voice come? Saul is under the impression he can see Samuel's ghost in the dark shadows. He insists. Feeling threatened, the witch explains that her voice is a relay between Samuel and him: "My King, I speak through my stomach which relates words to my throat, my lips are still." Ventriloquist and magic have been intimately interconnected since time immemorial.

From Sorcerer to Entertainer

Nothing much changed until the 17th century, when one can still find in the writings of the Italian anatomist, Fabrizio Aquapendente, this very odd diagnosis: "Ventriloquists are individuals with a well-articulated voice in their stomach and chest, the mouth and lips are closed. This is not natural, but magical and diabolical." The Church preferred to support a view of this nature than undertake serious research into this strange manifestation that seemed to have something to do with the voice of the soul.

Then came the *Encyclopédie* (the *Encyclopaedia*). At the end of the 18th century, the abbot Jean-Baptiste de La Chapelle, a French mathematician, contributor to the *Encyclopaedia*, ensured that henceforth, ventriloquism would be considered an art and a technique and no longer as a mysterious witches' practice. This citizen from Saint-Germain-en-Laye was obsessed with comprehending these phenomena. He was desperate to know how vowels can form without the lips moving and how ventriloquists manage to split their personality. His obstinacy dated back to an evening at which a ventriloquist show had fascinated him.

On February 17, 1770, Monsieur de Saint Gilles, aware of the abbot's keen interest in ventriloquism, invited him to accompany him to the back room of a merchant's shop, not far from the Château de Saint Germain. La Chapelle's eyes were riveted on Monsieur de Saint Gilles, who started off by telling funny stories. Then he went quiet, looked up at the ceiling, and suddenly a distant, very distant voice was heard calling "Father de La Chapelle!" The latter remained transfixed; in turn, he stared up at the ceiling, before enquiring, "Is that you?" The answer was obvious, yet the abbot remained doubtful. A few seconds passed; then again, one could hear, "No, don't look there, look over here!" The abbot looked down. His stupefaction was at its peak. This time, the voice seemed to be coming from the floorboards. Yet Monsieur de Saint-Gilles's lips hadn't moved. Only his impenetrable face seemed to follow the vibrations of his voice. This encounter marked Father La Chapelle for life.

On March 20 of the same year, another ventriloquist, Baron Mengen, hailing from Austria, met Father La Chapelle and engaged before him in what already then looked like a comic sketch. The Baron had a little ragdoll in his pocket with which he engaged in conversation: "You've given me rather disappointing news." To which the doll answered, "Sir, calumny is always easy. —Now you're being argumentative, Miss. —Sir, attacking may not be condoned, but defending oneself is always excused. —Shut up!" retorted the Baron, who then returned the doll to his pocket. She wriggled and murmured in a choking and grouchy voice, "That is typical of men; because they're all brawn, they confuse authority with justice."

The ragdoll had just come to life, so much so that an Irish officer passing by launched himself at the Baron's pocket. New moans emanated from it, giving the impression that the figurine was being choked and squashed. The officer let go, as if the figurine were a wounded animal. The Baron then showed the young officer that it was only a ragdoll, a common stick covered with cloth in lieu of a coat. The illusion was perfect. The Baron's lips hadn't moved, and his face showed compassion for his doll. The vivacity of the repartees between the ragdoll and the Baron had reinforced the illusion of magic.

The Baron produced two types of voice here. The first, when the doll was in the open pocket, was a near voice. The second, when the pocket was closed, was a distant voice.

How is such a phenomenon possible? People evoke the lips, the teeth, the esophagus; there is talk of a gift. When asked for his own explanation, the Baron seemed to find all this quite normal. For him, it was simply a voice that tricked people. His figurine allowed him to say things he couldn't say in a personal capacity and gave him the right to be impertinent.

His left hand held the doll and he formed his voice between his cheeks, tongue, and teeth, without having the impression that his stomach and abdomen had to make any particular effort or articulate a sound. He insisted on the lingual mobility, breathing, and rhythm he imposed on himself to kick off the dialogue with his doll.

In those days, analyzing this vocal mechanism was near impossible, as no instrument was capable then of observing the voice during the vocal utterances of a ventriloquist.

In 1876, the fascination with this phenomenon was running at its highest, when Fred Nieman performed with seven puppets. His own voice answered and chatted with the seven characters he had created. On stage, his agility as he passed from one voice to the next left everyone speechless. He mystified, amused, distracted, and intrigued. With him, the public entered a new dimension.

Vocal Alter Ego

We're in Paris, at the present time. The ventriloquist Christian Gabriel, whom I've enjoined to come so that I may understand the mystery of his art, enters my office. He discovered his gift of ventriloquism in his childhood. I would like to know how his puppet, Freddy, his inseparable, mischievous little monkey and alter ego, came about. Christian is very intimidated at the thought of putting his "double voice" on display in the office of a laryngologist, but it is Freddy who cuts in: "Are you going to hurt him?" There was no beating about the bush. Whom should I answer? "No, I won't hurt him. But don't you need to warm up your voice, Christian? —He doesn't need to," Freddy answers, nodding his head. Time to get to it. I introduce the video endoscope in the nasal fossa, down into the back of the throat, behind the uvula, and down to the roof of the larynx. This is the only way for me to get to the mechanisms that come into play during ventriloquism! By not introducing anything into the mouth, one avoids disturbing the movement of the lips, of the tongue, of the jaw, or of the pharyngeal muscles; he can therefore talk or sing, cough or laugh, with total freedom.

Freddy, the little stuffed chimpanzee with the cute look, takes his part very seriously, almost like a patient. Christian, the master of ceremony, animates Freddy's voice and, of course, his own. When Christian makes Freddy speak, he lends him his own voice. The contraction of his abdominal muscles meanwhile is visible.

In a same exhale, one can hear both Freddy's voice and Christian's voice. I'm struck by the speed of their repartee. It almost seems as if they're talking at the same time. The fact that both voices are produced on the same exhale gives the impression that there are no pauses between these two voices. The illusion is perfect. We really have the feeling that they are two people. This avalanche of words, these gestures, Christian's still lips, always slightly parted when Freddy intercedes and naturally mobile when his voice comes on, all this requires exceptional respiratory and pharyngeal-laryngeal efforts.

When Freddy talks, Christian has to force his voice intensely. His Adam's apple seems blocked. The little bone above it, the hyoid, is practically stuck under the mandible. The small muscle between the thyroid cartilage and the cricoid, that bony ring under the Adam's apple, contracts, thus helping the larynx to rise. All the neck muscles are tensed up. When Christian's voice comes on, they relax and find their natural position again.

In his throat, all the muscles are put to work; the pharyngeal muscles, the lateral muscles of the soft palate, and the uvula play a predominant role. They tighten up, taking on the shape of a pharyngo-laryngeal tube. The tongue is the orchestra leader. It has three parts: the apex or tip, the body, and the root. The body of the tongue lightly brushes the soft palate without ever making contact. When Freddy produces consonants, the tip of the tongue approaches the front teeth without touching them; a couple of millimeters separate them. Thus, sound is produced through the nose or the mouth by changing the course of the vocal emission and by accentuating the ventriloquist's illusionary skills. It is the phenomenon known as misdirection. This perfect synchronization happens in a record time: 1/10th to 1/15th of a second. When Christian speaks, the larynx returns to its initial position and its inverted cone shape. The tongue returns to its place, well in the center, no longer "pulling" the larynx upward. The lips now move normally.

Modern techniques for observing the larynx using video endoscopy and 3D imaging have enabled a better understanding of the workings of the muscles, joints, and bones of the vocal apparatus. Everything, or nearly everything, is visible. The muscular contractions deep in the tongue and also in the pharynx and soft palate down to the lips demonstrate the muscular strength required of a ventriloquist. Three-dimensional imagery reveals the agility of the laryngeal joint and the speedy response of the muscle between the thyroid and cricoid cartilages, which allow him to pass from Freddy's voice to Christian's voice. This changeover also enlists the hyoid bone, situated under the chin, from whence the heads of the lingual muscles and the muscles running from the hyoid to the larynx rise up. Thanks to their remarkable scanners and MRI machines, two doctors, Albert Castro and Rodolph Gombergh, brought to light in detail one of the fundamental characteristics of the ventriloquist: By virtue of the athletic strength of his neck muscles, he is a contortionist of the larynx.

Going deeper with the video endoscope, I notice the vocal cords are hard to make out, hidden by the muscle mass of the pharyngeal resonators. The vocal cords are vibrating. The only difference is that when Christian is on, the vocal cords lengthen, which is to be expected, since the puppet talks in a more highly pitched voice. When Freddy comes on, Christian passes from a chest voice to a head voice and the larynx tips up. This change in vocal register is accompanied by a complete change of attitude of the artist, and the physical silhouette of the voice changes when he passes from one voice to the other. A spectrograph enables us to analyze the speed at which he passes from a head voice to a chest voice. Two spectral identities become distinct. In a few fifteenths of a second, two voices clash and answer each other, yet both are produced by the same instrument: the larynx and only the larynx.

When Freddy speaks, the diaphragm is perfectly controlled, and the exhale is slow, lasting over 15 seconds, which allows the voice to be modulated, but more than that, it gives the ventriloquist time to put in place the muscles of the resonators that will shape the second voice. When Christian comes on, the phonatory exhale lasts seven to 10 seconds, which is normal.

The ventriloquist doesn't force his voice; he has the muscle resistance of an athlete.

We know the larynx is the source of vibration. But more is needed to produce vowels and consonants. The resonance box transforms itself, allowing the magic to operate. The production of vowels and consonants depends not only on the shape of the bucco-pharyngeal space but also on fast neurological control over this space and on lung capacity. The ventriloquist gives the impression he has created pseudo-lips behind his lips. This is very difficult to do, the more so since certain vowels and consonants are fearfully difficult to pronounce with only slightly parted lips. This vocal contortionist has to be foxy with letters, and it is the auditor who unconsciously completes the letter missing in a word. There is an alchemy operating here between the mechanics and word creation, with the interference of the linguistic brain. Others replace certain words; these gymnastics of enunciation are an impressive and cortical exploit by ventriloquists, who have to master what amounts to a second language. The auditor's left hemisphere understands and decrypts words that may not have been pronounced by the ventriloquist. When the latter says "Hexico," the audience hears "Mexico." Indeed, certain phonemes require that we close and move the lips, phonemes such as M, F, or P, which ventriloquists can't afford to do. The confidence trick here is sublime. What is important is not what is understood but what is heard.

Christian immobilizes his lips against his teeth when Freddy comes on. For the common man, teeth play a significant role in enunciation, and this is even truer of ventriloquists, for whom dental articulation is capital. Some of them clamp down hard on a pipe to facilitate ventriloquism.

The naked eye has a hard time observing and explaining the phenomenon of ventriloquism. Our eyes and our ears scrutinize the puppet or the ventriloquist, never both at the same time. If you want to catch a ventriloquist out in the subtleties of his art, it needs to be when he switches from his own voice to the puppet's voice.

We're so concentrated on what the ventriloquist says that we make it easy for him to pull the wool over our eyes. In the ventriloquist's art, seeing and hearing may be disjointed, but they dovetail perfectly. In a few tenths of a second, we pass from the puppet to the artist.

The artist is at the peak of his art when there is harmony between his gestures and his *voices*. The spectators' eyes are directed, guided, and controlled even by the artist's eyes. Their hearing is mistaken, its reaction not fast enough or precise enough. In trying to identify the exact origin of the voice, they have to watch the puppet or its master alternately, which adds to the magic of their inadequate acoustic perception.

When we talk normally, our lips move. When you speak, I watch you and I associate the movement of your lips with what you're saying to me. I conclude that the sounds I hear come from you. But the ventriloquist's voice is so fast that neither your eye nor your ears can locate it. Indeed, it is with our eyes that we try to make out the trajectory of acoustic waves. It is "the eyes that hear" and not our ears! The ventriloquist knows this, and he transforms his puppet into a bona fide actor that the spectator watches and consequently believes he can hear. The duo quickly turns into a three-way game with the public.

The spectators are hoodwinked, the more so because the puppet addresses itself directly to them. The magician of the voice has won the round. The trio of puppet/ventriloquist/spectator works.

Christian, during his performance, extends his visual field. When he animates Freddy, the puppet's stage presence and mobility are such that his master seems to have eyes behind his head! Other professionals I have talked with, such as James Hodges, Ronn Lucas, Jeff Dunham, and Valentine Vox in Las Vegas, whose publications are classics in this field, have also noted this idiosyncrasy.

Through his voice, the ventriloquist endows his puppet with emotion, gives it a personality. Every puppet has its own voice! Changes of tone, laughter, and tears animate the game that ensues between the ventriloquist and his double. When Freddy and Christian begin to dialogue, the spectators are enthralled. And I would say that Christian himself isn't far off believing in his own illusion.

The Show Is in the Audience

April 2001, Las Vegas. Toward evening, I arrive at the hotel where the world congress of ventriloquists is taking place where I witness a mind-blowing performance by the ventriloquist Jeff Dunham: three characters and voices from beyond the grave. The next day, around 10 a.m., I give a conference presenation. I'm the one on stage and they're my audience; for once the roles are reversed. My audience is very focused. I present the scientific aspects of the ventriloquism phenomenon, with supporting images and films. To my great delight, they're not put off by the medical and anatomical discourse. On the contrary, they seem highly interested and intrigued. They seem to be finding answers to questions some of them had entertained for too long.

After my contribution, Valentine Vox, the organizer of the congress who had invited me, opened the discussion to the floor. Astonishment! Nearly all participants produce a puppet. In a few seconds, the audience has doubled to 1,800 people! Everyone wants their puppet to ask a question, since the puppet knows no restrictions; after all, it isn't the ventriloquist talking. A Mexican man hiding behind his puppet launches the first question: "Chico Senior, my long-standing friend, has been a ventriloquist since childhood. Is that a gift?" Even if the gift manifests later, predispositions exist. I add that ventriloquism must be learned very young to potentiate not only the cerebral activation but also the training of the larynx. If you wanted a really accurate description, I would say that the ventriloquist is like a professional interpreter who masters two languages perfectly. Indeed, in a conference or a live televised retransmission, interpreters listen to what is said and, within a few tenths of a second, translate it simultaneously. They direct their brain in two directions: reception and emission, with a very short latency. This faculty demands constant practice. Beside their linguistic talents, these professionals have extraordinary powers of concentration. Is the same not true of ventriloquists? I should add that because of the resonators this vocal art requires, a good ventriloquist inevitability has to be over the age of puberty.

But imagine my surprise! At Chico's side, his 4.5-year-old son is already a ventriloquist. Chico Junior addresses me confidently through his puppet, Dumbo: "I'm Dumbo, and my master is the ventriloquist Chico Junior, who is, like his father, mother and grandfather before him, also a ventriloquist." The lips of the child haven't moved. I ask him to speak with his own voice. He sounds timid and somewhat hesitant. What duality in one so young! But think back: When we were kids, did we not make our toys speak? Was it not a form of liberation for us?

The questions from the audience start, but nearly all of them are posed by a puppet and not by the ventriloquist himself! I did not have 900 participants but 1,800. It was surreal. All these ventriloquists, from China, India, Japan, the United States, Germany, Belgium, or France, whom I was lucky enough to meet, had started to fashion their gift between the ages of 5 and 10. Most of them came from a circus or magician background. Ventriloquism is like medicine, singing, or stage comedy. It isn't a profession; it is a passion. These are not people who have a career in order to live; these are people who live for their career! In the ventriloquists' universe, the power of the voice is their life purpose.

After the conferences, the ventriloquists allow me to see them preparing themselves for their gala. In the wings of the stage, Christian, whom I meet again, spends 10 minutes warming his voice by voicing with his mouth closed. He vocalizes, practices yawning to stretch and warm up the muscles in his neck, and loosens his cervical vertebras, abdominal muscles, and resonator. He practices inhaling and exhaling deeply and relaxes the wrist and fingers that he will use to animate the puppet. Such is the ventriloquist's indispensable warm-up protocol before a show. Warm up and hydrate the voice, then the voice of the accomplice or accomplices, in order to avoid a mishap or an accident, such as a pulled vocal cord.

That night in Las Vegas, it was a timeless show that a restricted audience of some 200 people witnessed in that temple of ventriloquism. On stage, two ventriloquism techniques confront each other; one is a near voice or proximal voice, and the other is a distant voice. The use of misdirection (diverting the spectator's attention) is at its climax.

My extensive knowledge of the anatomical aspects of ventriloquism didn't make the mystery pale for me. I was fascinated.

When the ventriloquist uses his near voice, he holds the puppet close by. The ventriloquist's voice seems to come from his neck, as if piercing the skin; it is a throat voice, a head voice. The operational mode for the distant voice is different. The ventriloquist curls his tongue inside his mouth to enable the sound to echo. He creates a buzz, a bumblebee, in other words a to-ing and fro-ing of the harmonics in the mouth cavity. His larynx is tipped up. The voice is muffled, breathy; it seems to come from elsewhere, from the depths of the abyss, from the ceiling, from the other side of the wall.

This technical prowess is crucial for both types of ventriloquism. Moreover, on stage this day, the ventriloquists put in place an exceptional game between them, the puppets, and this public of professionals who know all the tricks of the trade and yet get caught up in the illusion, are moved, laugh, and get fired up every time a new character intervenes. Then, suddenly, no more puppets! One of the ventriloquists looks up and cocks his head; his stage accomplice follows suit, and so does the audience. "Who is there?" he asks. His face sets and one hears: "It's me, I'm on the first floor." Everyone looks up at the ceiling. The voice magician is at the height of his art! I have the impression of being in the company of the abbot, Frère de la Chapelle, on a certain morning of February 1770.

These congresses of ventriloquists are so amazing that, even if we know the tricks, we still are fascinated. This fictional reenactment, called The Ventriloquists Convention, uses as its starting point a gathering of ventriloquists that takes place every year in Kentucky. The originality of the show derives from the fact that it features a group of nine ventriloquists and their puppets, whose objective is not to entertain but to showcase questions concerning their profession, questions that surface much broader issues. Although ventriloquism issues from an inner voice, it never ceases to give us pause for reflection and to inspire artists.

The Mimic

If the ventriloquist is the contortionist of the larynx, the mimic is the acrobat of the larynx.

He is the artist of the artists: a thousand voices from one same voice!

Long confined to the private sphere or to the cabaret, this illusionist of the voice gained wider popularity in the 1970s thanks to television and continues to know a growing success. Since Thierry Le Luron, who impersonated with equal talent whether he was speaking or singing, impersonators have won wide acclaim and have grown in numbers. Today, they fill theaters, animate television shows, chronicle current events on the radio or on television, and keep pushing the limits of their art ever further.

What is their secret? The larynx is the music instrument of the impersonator. Does he, like the ventriloquist, show certain peculiarities? Around 90% of the mimics I have examined have an asymmetrical larynx. The vocal cords are powerful, and the epiglottis modifies their vocal timbre; the ligaments between the epiglottis and the vocal cord joints fashion a laryngeal warhead I have called a vocal cathedral, one that is particularly powerful and that can adapt itself to any type of imitation. The joint system of the vocal cords is the anatomical orchestra leader of the impersonator. These muscles allow the mimic to juggle with his voice, emphasizing if necessary the laryngeal asymmetry if it wasn't there originally. The speed of execution and precise mobility of these impersonators are the hallmarks of athletes of the vocal apparatus. The joint of the vocal cords, which are of unequal length, is also impressively supple. The arytenoids pivot during certain imitations. This genetic predisposition, this acoustic talent, requires in-depth work to copy the voice, text, and body language of the person impersonated. Talent is the differentiating factor here. The desire to impersonate perfectly can be taken very far. Thus, certain impersonators have been known to develop nodules on their vocal cords as a result of imitating artists with raspy voices! To my surprise, I found from observing the impersonators I was lucky enough to accompany, and as far as I could verify, that their larynx generally adopts the physical characteristics of the person they impersonate.

This was true in the case of Veronic Dicaire, Laurent Gerra, Thierry Garcia, Nicolas Canteloup, and Michaël Gregorio. By stretching one of their vocal cords, they're able to create at will different harmonics and thus come closer to the artist they're mimicking. And to our delight, they switch voices with ease, impersonating Yves Montand, Garou, Céline Dion, Ray Charles, Louis Armstrong, or our politicians.

Michaël Gregorio is probably one of the greatest impersonators of the singing voice. When asked which is his "real" voice, he answers, "My 'real' voice is the voice you hear in each of my impersonations, just altered by the resonators. Deep down, I never get the feeling I'm impersonating, I feel that I'm interpreting, in the fullest sense of the word, what I perceive in an artist. I trust my inner ear and then I let external ears listen to my work, those of my close circle first, then those of the public, who at the end of the day, is the best judge of an impersonator's success."

Most of the time, these virtuosos put the power of their voice in the service of humor or satire. Comedians at heart, their originality consists of creating their own scenarios, whether spoken or sung. The songs or tunes that are mimicked are often caricatured. Mimics such as Michaël Gregorio, who consecrate themselves exclusively to spoken and sung impersonations with the sole concern of attaining perfection in the reenactment of a variety of voices, are rare indeed. Thus, Michaël is able to switch from the ethereal high tones of Mylène Farmer to the gravelly bass of Louis Armstrong or Joe Cocker.

And yet, impersonators never lose their own personality and don't become a clone; they become a master interpreter, such as Laurent Gerra, or caricaturists such as Nicolas Canteloup or Thierry Garcia, who slightly exaggerate a trait. They don't become the other, which would be dangerous for their mental health and, like Faust, would spell their self-destruction. They preserve their own vocal identity. Fans of this art form always know which impersonator is at work. These three interpreters keep their own specific vocal harmonics while rendering a perfectly recognizable impersonation.

This gift of mimicry is inseparable from the gift of listening. The impersonator is able to hear himself and to recognize the landscape of his own voice, which most people are incapable of. Why do we have reticence to listen to our recorded voice? Well, most of the time, not only do we not recognize but we also don't like it. When we utter a sentence, we hear it both through the internal circuit of our body (our voice sends acoustic signals to our inner ear) and through our external circuit, which travels through the auricle of the ear and the external auditory canal (this is the only voice others hear). That is why we don't recognize our own voice; on a recording, our voice loses the low registers that our body had amplified because our bones only resonate to low pitches. So our voice comes across as shriller, less warm. We don't like it! The impersonator, on the other hand, has access to his external voice because he is able to more or less wipe out his internal voice; he hears himself speak just like you hear him. This means he can modulate his voice ad lib and re-create the timbre of the voice he seeks to impersonate. This fine detective of acoustics keeps his own personality, his own vocal identity, to which he adds the words, rhythms, tics, gestures, and even silences of the people he imitates.

The Castrati

Ventriloquists and impersonators, all acrobats of the voice, have in common that they put their voice on show by cultivating a certain vocal confusion, even inverting genders. An impersonator will quite often take on the voice of the opposite sex. The pursuit of this ambiguity is evident in many vocal traditions. In the West, the voice of the castrati illustrated this already in the baroque period: men with a woman's voice or, rather, a child's voice.

These artists, who left their mark on the lyrical arts in their day, have never ceased to be an influence since the 16th century, as witnessed by today's counter-tenor voices.

The nobility, the common folk, and the Church alike admired the castrati. Their feminine voice, powerful and resonant, stirred the enthusiasm of the crowds. The first castrati sang in the Sistine Chapel in 1562; Alessandro Moreschi was the last of the castrati to perform there in 1903, just before Pope Leo XIII formally forbade the presence of castrati in the Church for good. As much in demand for singing sacred chants as for singing profane music and opera, they owe their Golden Age and the durable popularity of the power of their voice, to which they sacrificed their life, to the following episode.

In 1688, the Duke of Mantua was in Rome, where he attended high mass, invited by Pope Innocent XI. That same evening, he attended a concert given by the singer Georgina, accompanied by castrati. He succumbed to the charm of her sensual voice, and when asked by the pope what he most appreciated in Rome, he answered it was the singer Georgina. Angered by his answer, the pope demanded the exile or banishment to a convent of all female singers and, furthermore, forbade all women from singing or appearing on stage. Georgina was lucky enough to escape when the pope's henchmen came to arrest her. Pope Clement XI later extended this prohibition, initially restricted to Rome, to the whole of Christendom, who decreed, "No person of the feminine gender is allowed to learn music with the intention of using her musical knowledge to become a singer. Indeed, one knows that a beautiful woman singing on stage, yet purporting to preserve her virtue, can be likened to someone aspiring to jump into the Tiber River without wetting his feet." This prohibition went a lot further than Saint Paul's: "*Molieres taceat in ecclesia*," literally "Women shall be quiet in Church," which effectively forbade women from singing in churches. Ipso facto, chanting being an indispensable religious prop, the door was now wide open for castrati to triumph.

The West discovered the first castrati in the 15th century. Hailing from the Orient, they made a name for themselves in the Church where Gregorian chanting required such a high register that few singers could aspire to it. Moreover, it required a perfect mastery of elocution, since the higher the register, the more difficult it became to pronounce the words. These highly unusual, asexual voices with a high tessitura were hard to find. Falsetto voices were too expensive to hire, as were the castrati from Spain. Hence, in 1592, Pope Clement VIII encouraged the castration of young boys, so that as adults, they might retain their angelic voice, with a very high pitch and plenty of amplitude. Initially hired to sing exclusively liturgical music, the castrati were soon also in demand in the opera.

Farinelli's renown has survived the passing of centuries. His real name was Carlo Broschi and he was born on January 24, 1705, near Bari, which back then still belonged to the province of Naples. Trained in Naples by the illustrious Porpora, he became a leading lyrical voice in Europe, spending 25 years at the court of the king of Spain, Philip V, and owed his extraordinary success to the mind-blowing range of his register, which covered nearly five octaves. Why he was castrated has never been formally established. There was talk that it was due to a riding accident or that it was a deliberate choice his father made to preserve the boy's naturally exceptional soprano voice. Furthermore, cupidity can't be totally ruled out as one of his father's motivations, since the castrati, considered like stars, earned a lot of money. In any case, Carlo Broschi became Farinelli.

The voice is under the influence of sex hormones, androgens in the case of men and estrogens and progesterone in the case of women. Androgens influence specific organs to provoke their masculinization through sexual characteristics affecting hairiness, the genitals, and the voice. At puberty, androgens and especially testosterone trigger the masculinization of the adolescent and the development of the Adam's apple and a man's voice, the voice breaks and becomes more manly. Testosterone facilitates and increases the hypertrophy of muscles such as the biceps and, consequently, also the muscles of the vocal cords. The child's voice will remain feminine, angelic, and asexual, but only as long as the child is castrated before puberty. If done after puberty, castration will have no influence on the voice, which remains masculine due to important secretions of testosterone at this stage of a young boy's life, secretions that have a definitive impact on the muscles and cartilages of the body.

How is it that despite an absence of male hormones, the castrato is nevertheless able to develop a powerful male voice and an intensity and lung capacity that seem at odds with the high notes he can reach? In fact, though testosterone no longer has an impact on the castrato, he retains a hormonal environment linked to the

XY chromosome and made up of a number of nonsexual hormones—namely, thyroid, corticosteroid, and growth hormones. Due to the absence of testosterone, the pharynx and larynx are finely muscled. Since men have more secretions of thyroid and growth hormones than women do, these hormones come into their own again: XY and XX. These hormones have nothing to do with the testicles but with the specific glands that contribute to the energy, power, and build of the castrato.

The partial castration of the castrati wasn't the emasculation that eunuchs underwent. The technique was well oiled. In principle, it was undertaken only if the child and his singing master agreed to it. It consisted of annihilating the testicles—in other words, ensuring that they would no longer secrete male hormones. The child was drugged and placed in a hot bath to numb him. An incision was made just above the testicles, and then the spermatic cords were tied, with their spermatic canal, but also their arteries and testicular veins. This ensured a rapid necrosis of the testicles. The necrosis could be partial, and thus certain castrati could still have an erection and were proud of their unaffected libido, although they weren't allowed to marry and had, according to Pope Clement VIII, pledged their voice to the Kingdom of God. From this castration resulted a hybrid individual, with the energy and looks of a man but the long, fine muscles of a woman and sometimes gynoid looking (i.e., with a woman's pear shape).

A prodigy of vocal technique, Farinelli had a falsetto or counter-tenor voice. Castration had enabled him to keep his soprano voice, and since his vocal register had a very broad range, he could sing a succession of trills and cascades and pass from the lowest pitch to the highest with disconcerting speed. He could also sustain a note for almost two minutes with apparent ease, whereas a professional singer can rarely hold a note for longer than 45 seconds. Thanks to his laryngeal, thoracic, and auditory anatomical predispositions, his pneumophonic loop (breathing and vocal cords) and audio-phonatory loop (hearing and retrocontrol of the voice) were outstanding. The power and capacity of his lungs were impressive. His resonators also benefited from these hormonal secretions, giving rise to bewitching harmonics. Is the presence of low-pitched harmonics, overlaid with high-pitched harmonics, not what renders singing beautiful? An amazing soprano voice needs superb high notes, but the bass notes hone the vocal landscape. Is the beauty of a diamond not set off by its jewelry case? Similarly, a bass singer needs high tones if he is to fully develop the powers of seduction of his tessitura.

Giovenale Sacchi, musicologist and contemporary of Farinelli, describes Farinelli's triumphal beginnings thus: "Farinelli is to sing with a virtuoso trumpet player. It is clear a duel has been staged between a wind instrument, the trumpet player, and a wind and cord instrument, the larynx. The public holds its breath, expectant. The two artists are about to confront each other. The melody begins with a note held in *fermata*. The trumpet begins the note softly, holds it from *pianissimo* to *fortissimo* for so long that the public is beside itself. No one believes that Farinelli, despite his talent, will manage to hold this note that long! His turn comes. He also starts off *pianissimo*, his voice crystalline and natural. He holds it for so long that it unleashes explosive applause and cries of admiration. But Farinelli goes further. He sings the musical phrase again and adds brilliant trills to it that no one before him has ever attempted. A vocal genius was born."

The castrato is hostage to the power of his voice. He enjoys no freedom. His life is dedicated to his art. Are castrati not talked of as "a third gender"? How many children have been sacrificed to get one Farinelli? Future castrati worked their voices 10 hours a day and their career started after they were castrated between the ages of eight and 10. The castrato is nothing less than a "vocal monster"! Farinelli sacrificed his body for his voice. He forced his public to question the accepted points of reference for a man's voice and a woman's voice. He could sing a *legato*, that smooth Bel Canto string of lengthened notes, to perfection. He also played with the fullness of his voice, putting his remarkable power in the service of a *vibrato* that could last several dozen seconds. I should point out, however, that today, all these characteristics can often be observed in singers, be they lyrical or variety artists—Céline Dion's *belting* being a good example of this.

The public's infatuation with Farinelli was reenacted thanks to a film by Gérard Corbiau, released in 1994. The film director turned to the institute for acoustic/musical research and coordination (IRCAM) at the postproduction stage to re-create the castrato's voice. Technical prowess was needed to render a realistic impression of this lost voice. Corbiau created Farinelli's voice by fusing two voices together. The voices of the American counter-tenor Derek Lee Ragin and the Polish coloratura Ewa Mallaz Godlewska were mixed. It was a genius association. But it turned out to be an unbelievable association, not least because it was surprisingly contrary to expectation. The high-pitched voice was sung by the counter-tenor and the low voice by the soprano! Thanks to this preternatural voice, the 18th-century miracle was born again and the film was a hit with the public, suggesting that its fascination for these extreme and unclassifiable voices had never paled. The exhilaration of seduction, the allurement of vibrations, the spell of harmonics, such was the power of the voice of the castrato.

The Voice Is an Unfinished Symphony

The voice, light of our thoughts, is the paintbrush of our soul. For you and me, the voice is both the motor and the immediate and immanent projection of our conscience.

Each voice is an orchestration in which we are orchestra leader and musician, actor, and spectator. We decide what the tone will be, the mode, major or minor, the color or expression, the tempo—adagio, allegro, or presto. Slow or fast, the rhythm is specific to each of us. Often synchronized with others, sometimes offbeat, it can also play solo. These rhythmical patterns are two-time and three-time beats. Like man's heart, the rhythm can become anarchical, with extrasystoles, and go into arrhythmia. It is the rhythm of anger, on the edge when we voice our stress, music with no logic in its rhythmicity. The extrasystoles of the voice remind one of a child hammering on the keyboard of a piano in a disorderly, anarchical, discordant manner, a noise accompanying a voice, not a voice accompanying a noise.

The height of one's register is structured within a vocal tessitura that is our own. Our voice is a symphony, our words its composition. The symphony of the voice varies across cultures.

In Italy, bedrock of the Bel Canto, the language itself is like music. When an Italian speaks, vowels sing. The music and language of India range over other harmonics with improvisation rules. The frequencies used may offend our ears. Their consonance and dissonance are unsettling. They're in the eighth tone or in a quarter tone above or below the designated pitch, which we don't use. And yet that language, that music has its own words, its own vibratos, rhythms, and flourishes. The unsettling effect on me of these bizarre harmonics brought home to me their importance. They're essential to the landscape of these languages. The richness of our culture is born from our differences. The mix has embellished the melody of our spoken and sung voice.

But in the days of Plato or Victor Hugo, people took the time to listen to others, for fear their "knowledge" might dissipate. The podcast hadn't been invented yet.

In the old days, the slower tempo of people's lives was influenced by their environment, by the time it took to get around, the slow pace of information. Communication was in harmony with those times. Nowadays, technical advances in transportation, in the media, and in acoustic communications have imposed an out-and-out race on our vocal expression. The voice has left behind its flourishes, its courtesy trimmings and niceties. Utterances become harsh, sometimes as cutting as a staccato. People stick to essentials or what the individual considers essential: "Good day Madam, how are you and how is your family?" has become "Hi, what's up?" The rapper, whose shortened silences re-create a remarkable rhythm in the spoken voice by playing around with every syllable, has replaced the crooner Frank Sinatra. Amazing techniques may have propelled orchestration and musical and vocal arrangements into another dimension, but the voice is still the voice, whatever the technology. It is a symphonic script that is personal and that manifests its power whatever the height of the note. The higher it is, the more high-handed it seems; the deeper it is, the more reassuring and even imposing it is. But that isn't enough. Let us now add a rhythmic value to every note and thus be able to determine a cadence, as on a sheet of music. The closed note figure in black on a musical score is the unit of time. Talking in quarter notes is very different from talking in sixteenth notes: "Let me tell you" is different from "Let me—tell you."

"Music is the silence between the notes," Debussy was fond of saying. And Miles Davis seemed to echo these words: "The real music is in the silences, the notes just dress these up." Thus, the figure of silence, signaled by a pause or a quarter-note in a partition, corresponds not only to the breathing cadence in the spoken or sung voice but also in each of us the hallmark of our charisma, of our seductiveness, of our vocal signature. I shall come back to this.

The Voice Is a Work of Art

The voice is a work of art. It plays with the colors of words, with the harmonics of vibrations and with the silences that make us stop and think. That silence, the one that screams at you, that seduces you, that insists on having your attention, is what gives the voice its strength. The voice inscribes itself in a present time that prepares the future in the shadows of the past.

Having been passionate about laryngology and the virtuosos of the larynx for 30 years, I now know for sure that the voice is a work of art. Armand Drouant, the famous art merchant, attributes a value to a work of art on the basis of five qualities: its sincerity, its sonority, its color, its style (the originality of the concepts), and its polish (the originality of execution). The same appraisal scale can be applied to the voice. In this case, style and polish can be considered to be the signature of the voice. If one of these five qualities were lacking, the power of the voice would be undermined.

The voice isn't material; it isn't like clay that can be molded or like a diamond that can be cut. It is like the light, intangible, elusive, and immaterial. It is invisible, and yet it possesses wavelengths and a vocal specter. Like the light, it travels through a prism, the prism of our emotions. The voice is sculpted by its timbre, its rhythm, its prosody. Just as Michelangelo professed that he didn't sculpt stone, he undressed it, the voice undresses our soul. It is dynamic, on the move, volatile, no sooner expressed; it already belongs to the past. Gone in an instant, it is the instant. If a photo immortalizes the present, the voice vibrates the present. But the voice is an instrument that tunes into others. We talk or sing for and thanks to someone, for and thanks to a public. The person listening stimulates or inhibits the vocal genius and virtuosity of the artist of the voice, galvanizes and animates the artist's vocal creation. A vocal signature is as much the other person as it is the self; it's an alchemy so tricky that striving for it can threaten the voice with parasite phenomena that are well known to voice performers and that may compromise and debilitate the power of this voice.

Stage Fright and Stress

Stage fright, this irrational fear that strikes one just before coming on stage, has many psychological causes. It can be brought on by simple superstition, by the fear that we won't be good enough or by any anxious anticipation, by an unfortunate cat-whistle at a previous performance, and so on. Stage fright is an element of stress that has a distinctive feature. It can't exist in the absence of a public, even if the public is just one person.

The magnetic atmosphere of a show shouldn't be underrated. Indeed, the bad vibes sent by just two or three hostile spectators in the public are enough to destabilize the artist and affect his vocal performance. This is why I often advise voice professionals who consult me to invite at least one friend to the show on opening night, who will be a positive and reassuring presence in the audience. The artist just has to look his way from time to time to benefit from a positive transfer of emotional energy.

Stress triggers an impressive number of physical and mental manifestations. The most striking of these is a super-fast hormonal response. In the case of say adrenaline or cortisol, the response time is in tenths of seconds.

Too much stress may sometimes trigger a vagal attack, a cold sweat, excessive salivation, diarrhea, or a slower heartbeat.

There are two stages of stress. The first stage is an alert phase. This is often positive stress, the sort we've all experienced when we have to speak in public, sit for an oral exam, or prepare for a sporting event. The brain captures the signal ("Be attentive, it's show time!"). The center of emotion, the hypothalamus, is stimulated, releasing adrenaline, which is both a hormone and a neurotransmitter. Stimulated by stress, it causes the heart rate to speed up and increases blood pressure. It provokes anxiety and dryness of the mouth and throat. The pupils dilate and our hearing becomes more acute. The brain, better oxygenated, is now hyper alert, vigilant, ready to react. Internal strength is at its maximal. A fight or flight response can be immediate. At times, the adrenaline is over the top. We get tension headaches and gastric reflux with an excess of hydrochloric acid in the stomach. Digestion slows down. The second phase is one of endurance. It kicks off when stress persists and accompanies action. This phase is also good stress. Cortisol is stimulated. Like adrenaline, it is secreted by the adrenal glands. Cortisol's job is simple: to maintain a constant level of sugar in the blood in order to conserve our cardiac, cerebral, and muscular energy. Indeed, our brain burns 20% of the body's sugar in action. So adrenaline is the body's response to an emergency; it's like the intensive care unit of our body. And cortisol is its resistance, its endurance.

Come and See the Comedians

The voice of the comedian, actor, or singer is the interface between the performer and his public. He has to inhabit a text that he invests with emotion while considered by spectators to be the incarnation of that text. This carnal emotion is the paradox of the artist's voice.

If the performance is to seem sincere, the first step is to learn the text by rote in order to "forget it" and then repossess it. Although repetition is necessary, playing the text on stage like a translation is fatal. Playing it out of habit destroys all spontaneity. The vocal landscape blurs, and the voice becomes an affective desert and loses its power.

Victorio Gassman told me, in the 1990s, that when an actor is chosen for a role, he needs to be not only in harmony with the text but also with his body language. Moreover, the theater imposes a real constraint in that a simple "hello" has to be heard as clearly from the back row as from the front. The very exacting school of Charles Dullin taught you how to place your voice without forcing, how to forge your vocal mechanics, how to master interpretation. The voice alone is not enough; talent is indispensable. Everybody has a gift: talent is to make working very hard your gift. Some of his students practiced for hours on end, seeking to find the right note that would give the illusion of reality. Others would run the risk of improvising, which goes to show that the talent and experience of an artist, as projected by the stamp of the voice, can take different paths. But we must not forget what Beethoven used to say: "To play a wrong note is not important but to play without your heart is unpardonable."

I was lucky to meet many artists throughout my career, such as Anthony Quinn and Robert Hossein. Both have seductive, pleasant voices thanks to their harmonics, light veils, and vibratory mystery. He went through life without losing any of the character of his voice or its very particular grain. Out of his imperfections, the artist manages to bring forth emotion. Though his larynx presents certain distinctive features comparable to those of Garou, the irreplaceable hunchback Quasimodo in the musical comedy *Notre-Dame de Paris*, both are men who put their vocal power in the service of their creativity. Voices that seduce are those of well-known performers such as Laureen Bacall, Humphrey Bogart, John Wayne, or Henry Fonda, lightly veiled, stroking the ear without ever offending it, a voice that soothes with a charm that defies description. One would recognize it anywhere; its distinctive signature would stand out even in a crowd, like the great voices of the stage and screen such as Yul Brynner or Charlton Heston.

Whether an actor is playing in a Shakespeare drama or in a play, his voice becomes a capacitor of the vibrations of his external world but also of his internal world. When on stage, the actor feeds off the collective; he gets his energy directly from the public, transforms it thanks to its emotional heritage, amplifies it, and sends it back to the public through his voice. The same happens with radio and television; they too are emotional amplifiers in which the voice, as an instrument of emotion, exerts a remarkable power over the auditor.

Cyrano de Bergerac

Despite having been for years a pillar of the TNP (the Théâtre National Populaire) of Jean Vilar and despite having performed in dozens of roles, Daniel Sorano will remain a legendary interpreter of Edmond Rostand's play *Cyrano de Bergerac*. Yet there have been many Cyranos in the history of the theater, with the greatest actors having played the role. Here the key word is really interpretation. With its famous monologue of the nose or its magnificent poems at Roxane's balcony when only the power of the voice exists, this play offers, like a color palette, a whole range of possible interpretations of the same text.

When the French comedian Gérard Depardieu plays Cyrano and when Daniel Sorano plays it, they both do it with their own signature. Both offer exceptional interpretations that trigger different emotions, different sensations, colors, and elucidations. In 1989, Gérard Depardieu, with his earthy nature, his strength, his energy, played a Cyrano who is a powerful swordsman, who has rhythm in his speech, whose tirades are clear and brilliant. The stage vibrates constantly in a cycle of calms and storms. In 1960, Daniel Sorano was an "ethereal" Cyrano, slim yet with a deep voice, whose sword work was like a ballet. Through his voice, which was all delicacy as it graduated from the red of passion to the blue of melancholy, he colored an acoustic world in which his emotion could be found in the subtlety of the harmonics. Had he not earned the nickname Sorano de Bergerac because of his remarkable identification with his part?

The *Cyrano* of Jean-Paul Belmondo oscillates between these two interpretations; he portrays elegant impertinence, plays with words and gestures, and impersonates eloquence. These three voices have three very different vocal signatures, and the reactions and feelings they trigger in the audience are so different that one could believe that the text, which never changes, has changed from one interpretation to the next: same words, three different translations.

This transition from the paper to the stage version of the play is beyond Edmond Rostand's control. The text of his *Cyrano de Bergerac* is sculpted like a work of art, but the stage performer "brings it to life." Such is the power of the voice.

Golden Gate, How Do You Do It?

In December 1988, during a gala evening, I heard Clyde Wright sing. A mixture of blues and gospel, the wonderful voice of this tenor of the Golden Gate captivates me. How does he manage to retain such deep harmonics while singing in tenor? How does he pull off sliding his voice from an impressively clear note to a velvet voice whose husky timbre recalls the voice of Louis Armstrong? At the end of the evening, I go to him, full of admiration, and ask him if he will let me see his voice. He stares at me in confusion, not understanding the meaning of my words. I explain that I am an ENT specialist, that the mysteries of the voice are my passion, and that video endoscopy allows me to film the vocal cords. Despite the late hour, I can't resist giving him a quick exposé on the larynx! He responds warmly and agrees to come by my office sometime in the next few days.

Observing his larynx, I'm impressed. In slow frame, the video endoscopy reveals to me very powerful vocal cords that vibrate symmetrically, as is to be expected in the case of a professional singer. Yet something isn't quite as usual in this larynx, though I can't put my finger on it. I view the images again and again. The larynx is certainly extremely supple. What else? In fact, this suppleness stems from the joint of each vocal cord. Instead of facing off each other, almost bumping into each other as is normal when the glottal space closes during phonation, Clyde's vocal cord joints slide against each other. And then I pierce the mystery. At the end of his voicing, when he sings the blues, one of the joints passes over the other one! Another particularity comes to light. The parts contiguous to and adjoining these joints vibrate when he sings in Louis Armstrong style, and this isn't at all usual. This is what makes Clyde Wright's vocal identity. But I want to go further. Is this vocal signature of the blues singer, of the gospel singer, specific to Clyde Wright, or is it fortuitous? Do the other singers of the Golden Gate Quartet have the same signature? I'm keen to film their vocal cords and ask him if they might come to see me.

The four singers of the Golden Gate agree to humor me. I examine them. The discovery I make is surprising. I admit I was even stupefied! My Sherlock Holmes magnifying glass is my video fibrolaryngoscopy; with it, I'm able to bare the secrets of this remarkable quartet. But before I brief them on my findings, Clyde Riddick takes the time to fill me in on the fascinating history of the group. In 1939, the group was singing in New York. Segregation reigned, yet white people were dancing to the tunes of Afro-Americans. Inadmissible! Then in 1941, Eleanor Roosevelt invited them to the White House, in Washington, for the investiture of President Roosevelt. To cut a long story short, it was in 1949, in Memphis, that Clyde Riddick met Elvis Presley, then barely 15, who said to him, "Clyde, I want to sing like you." The music of the Golden Gate Quartet had crossed generations. When I met them, Clyde Riddick, their first tenor, was over 80, as was Orlandus Wilson, baritone and founder of the Golden Gate. Anthony Gordon and of course Clyde Wright had integrated the group in 1954.

That January morning in 1988, all four were in my office. The laryngeal images of the quartet were now available for us to see, and surprise, all four singers showed the same sliding of the vocal cord joints I had observed in Clyde Wright. They exhibited the same laryngeal suppleness. Hence their vocal ranges. These legendary voices had allowed me to understand the vocal gymnastics of gospel and blues singers. Since then, I have examined several gospel and blues singers, and their vocal signature was no different. These warm and captivating unusual voices are able, when singing gospel songs, to inspire a congregation of faithful to greater spiritual heights. As Saint Augustin has said, "Singing is like praying twice."

It's true that nowadays, more than an instrument of prayer, the singing voice has become the perfect instrument of seduction. Young singers are the knights in shining armor of modern times. They compete in television shows before the entire nation. Their sword is their vocal vibration. This is a new kind of battle. These knights of the voice are athletes who expend themselves physically and who also bare their souls, which can be dangerous for them! Their arena is the media. The television viewers pronounce the sentence; these gladiators of the voice risk an affective trauma that could be fatal. However, I should qualify this comment by pointing out that in a show such as *The Voice*, these aspiring singers are judged by true professionals of the voice, whose verdict can at times seems harsh but is mostly fair and never humiliating.

Does a Professional Voice Profile Exists?

I may only be the instrument maker and repairman of the voice, but over time I gained the conviction that a good ENT specialist has to make a point of regularly listening to artists in their own environment if he is to understand these injured voices, these pure voices, these broken voices. Which is why outside of my professional activities and surgical interventions, I've always sought out the company of voice performers, and our discussions concerning the vocal arts have been a priceless school of life for me.

Ruggero Raimondi, an exceptional baritone whose limpid voice plays with high and low registers, revealed to me that though comfortable in the tenor and bass registers, he felt in perfect harmony with the baritone register. In classical singing, the tenor exhibits shorter vocal cords and often a stocky physique, whereas the baritone has longer cords, as well as a wider range of registers and a streamlined silhouette. Thanks to his laryngeal suppleness and his highly developed vocal cords, Ruggero Raimondi very rarely suffered from problems tied to voice forcing. I must add that his life hygiene meets the same high standards he sets himself, he who was "the" legendary baritone of *Don Giovanni* or *Boris Godounov*.

The register his larynx imposes on him binds a voice performer. Whereas in the high notes, one can always try to go that little bit higher, in the low notes, there is a bottom line that is impassable. Nature has its laws: The tenor, the baritone, the deep bass, the lyrical soprano, and the alto each present a distinctive conformation. The conformation of the vocal tube enables the creation of harmony. A lifetime is then spent trying to improve it. Thus, the artist's temperament is a determining factor in his career. His conviction and his passion will be dedicated to his vocal art.

In most cases, a singer's build is a clue to his vocal tessitura. The anatomy of the larynx, its structure, and its dimensions are often in relation to the build. The tenor is usually stocky, with a strong, well-muscled neck, especially at the back; his larynx is less angled, more roundly curved, the Adam's apple less prominent. His larynx is a laryngeal cone that is relatively short but with a wide base. The thyroid cartilage is less developed than in a baritone or a deep bass, and his cricothyroid membrane is very strong and short.

The bass singer is usually willowy. The laryngeal cone is deeper, the vocal cords long and powerful.

The baritone is often tall and slim, with a well-muscled neck. The larynx is also long and pointy, with marked angles, a prominent Adam's apple, and a large space between the cricoid ring and the thyroid cartilage. In terms of stature, the baritone is between the tenor and the bass.

These simplified descriptions have the merit of being clear, but they're oversimplistic. Among female singers, the morphological differences between sopranos and altos are hard to spot at first glance.

Voice performers who haven't had any formal singing or theatrical training are unaware of the importance of the stomach and perineum, unlike singers and comedians, who know their instrument well. Breathe with your stomach, we are told. The abdomen is padded with numerous muscles that help us breathe and keep the viscera supported, like strapping. But controlled breathing has to be learned and practiced, and voice performers are athletes in their own right.

Vincent's Story

Last November, I was a guest on a television set to give my expert opinion on certain singers who at some point in their career had "lost" their voice. The show was for the most part consecrated to the French singer C. Badi, a young singer I appreciate, and on this occasion, I met Vincent, whose story fascinated me, a story he has written about in a book and that, with his blessing, I shall tell here. Vincent is now 48. Twenty years earlier, he was just beginning a promising career in the opera as a tenor, when one day . . .

Vincent spent a great deal of his time traveling. One night, he would be singing in Peking, the next day in Karlsruhe, then filling in for another singer in Basel on the spur of the moment, and so it went. Under pressure from his agents, he lived in a whirlwind, under great emotional stress. Burnout followed. His voice cracked up. As is known, the tenor's voice has one of the highest tessituras. The tenor hits the high notes using his chest voice, which is risky and practically a tightrope balancing act. As at the circus, the public watches out for the tenor's high C.

Vincent didn't start out in life thinking of becoming a voice performer. It was while doing voluntary work in Burundi that he discovered his tenor's voice. Back in France, he took some singing lessons, which confirmed his singing potential. He remembers the only concert that his father came to hear him sing at, when he was starting out. It turned out to be one of the greatest moments of his life, because from that point on, he and his father, who knew he was fatally ill, enjoyed real communication, and he became aware of the power of his voice, of its effect, and of the good it could do to people around him. His father passed away the day after his opening night in Wagner's *Lohengrin*, in which Vincent, for the first time, was leading soloist. Obviously something powerful happened, similar to a rite of passage. He became more self-confident, to the point of acting recklessly. He confessed that it fed his ego, but he didn't know how to manage his energy well. Today, he recalls that his fast-track training (nine years condensed into three) meant his foundations were flawed, from both a technical and an emotional standpoint. At one time, he thought he had reached stardom and became less vigilant, which can be fatal in this profession. He had a red alert, which brought about the first interruption of his career.

In 2003, he returned to the stage in the role of Pelleas, a role in a register between baritone and tenor, with deep C notes that he wasn't used to singing. He wasn't ready for this part, which was too heavy emotionally for him. As a result, his low notes were muted, and he had to push to get them to ring out (all this without a microphone and accompanied by an orchestra of 100 musicians). The inevitable happened. He lost his voice, this time for good. The injury was serious enough to make his throat hemorrhage, accompanied by a feeling that his throat was blocked, fixed in stone forever. Indeed, he had to give up his stage career.

The significant part of Vincent's story is that he was pressured into singing lower than his natural tessitura. Forcing the voice in a low register causes muscle tears. A comparison would be asking a marathon runner to do a 100-meter sprint. Pushing the voice strains it; this is what I call an internal injury of the voice. Notwithstanding the mechanics of the voice, there is also the emotional aspect tied to the role-play; when both are ill-adapted for the part, as happened with Vincent, it's asking for trouble.

After a total rest of his voice for a month, Vincent's voice made a fairly speedy recovery. The nodule may have been small, but emotionally, he was a broken man. In 2004, at the age of 38, professionally he was dead in the water. He tried everything—a reputed ENT specialist, a voice clinic in Paris, auditions with an agent in New York to relaunch his career in North America—nothing worked. After dilapidating his parents' heritage, he was destitute, living in a tiny studio flat in the greater Paris. He was on the brink of becoming homeless. He touched rock bottom and at that point heard an inner voice, a shrill, child-like voice, the voice of little Vincent. He paid attention to his inner silence, as he explains. His little voice reminded him of his dreams: dreams of wolves, of Canada, of forests and Amerindians. He started to breathe again. Something inside of him was talking. A little flame came alight again. And he invested his last penny in a lifesaving trip to Canada.

There he relearned to live, to simply breathe in nature, to touch the trees, to live in the moment, to feel happy to be alive with no need for material frills. He felt his voice was back and maybe made the mistake of wanting to start over as before. But today wasn't yesterday. In the professional world of singing, you are soon old news. But more than that, he got an urge to create something that would meld his two passions in life, singing and nature. Hence the birth of his concept of lyrical hikes through the forest with the objective of reappropriating the five senses through song and acoustic vibrations in the midst of trees.

That day, on the television set, I felt no need to make a long discourse, preferring to leave the floor to Vincent, whose story seemed to me such a rich learning experience. It illustrated perfectly something I firmly believe in and that isn't brought up often enough in matters pertaining to the power of the voice: that inner voice, our silent voice, the one that accompanies us throughout our life, the one only we can hear. It is the matrix of the power of our audible voice. It is an essential and ever-present force giving impulsion to our projects, our actions, our decisions. The silent voice, the voice of the self to the self, the voice that catches up with us on the starting block as we're about to dive; this voice even stimulates the production of oxytocin, the hormone that has a significant impact on sports activities, as do endorphins. In the context of sporting events, this inner voice resonates in our head without any sound being audible; it has a power each of us knows perfectly, the power to reassure us, motivate us, give us momentum, and guide us.

CHAPTER 5

The Voices of Silence

André Dussollier once told me that at the end of one of his plays, he murmurs, in one of those theatrical murmurs that can be heard from the back row, "Yes, I cheated on you, but . . . " and he goes quiet. The audience holds its breath. Nothing. A few second later, still nothing. The audience is restless, hanging on the actor's lips, a vague muttering rises from the auditorium. The waiting becomes trying, and the audience is suddenly in doubt. What if the great André has forgotten his lines? "You see, Jean, it was the best way to bring them into my world." And how right he was! There's nothing like silence to put the voice on show.

I normally tell my clients that it is from their silences that I recognize their problems. However, that's not to say that all silences have the same meaning, especially not in politics. Silences are an extraordinary weapon, because they give the listener time to assimilate what has just been said and to appropriate it, repeating it silently.

The Strategy of Silences

In their discourses, politicians use pauses as a fundamental means of winning the audience over or of conserving power. But, and this is a capital point, remarkably defined by Danielle Duez of the CNRS (the French National Centre for Scientific Research): depending on the message to be delivered and of his position on the political chessboard, the speaker organizes his pauses and silences very differently. The challenger, the one wanting to take power, such as Jacques Chirac when he faced François Mitterrand in 1988, speaks fast, with rare pauses. The president in power has an easier time of it. His pauses, even his silences, are like barbs he uses against his adversary, his speech slow and self-confident. An explanation of his project is necessary but not indispensable. Above all, he needs to keep his cool, lead the opponent on without exposing himself, play the empathy card, and maintain a serene rhythm.

The way time is managed and distributed while we talk is a marker of the power of our voice. The voice can most definitely create a virtual space that is social, physical, and emotional. The vocal space can be intimate among close friends and glacial in a political discourse in which the voice is almost impersonal, each word well articulated, the delivery slow to allow the public to integrate the discourse. The musicality of the voice comes alive as the debate progresses, feeding off the person opposite, be it a journalist, a political opponent, or the public.

As for silence, it has a very symbolic role in our vocal voice, notably the silence that raises questions or is a warning sign. When the comedian, the politician, or Joe Blog stops talking, you hold your breath. That silence is so powerful, it leaves you "without voice."

Elsewhere, silence can be a mark of respect, whether in holy places, during commemorations, or during a minute of remembrance.

Nonetheless, silence needs to be subtly meted out. Too long, over four seconds, it may destabilize the auditor, who switches off, his mind ready to wander off. This is what actors refer to as "the Christmas tree" syndrome. The spectator ceases to focus on the action and thinks about the feast awaiting him after the show.

Some individuals are able to draw advantage from this propensity that silence has to make us dream, just before boredom sets in. "I have a dream . . . " Martin Luther King Jr.'s famous speech on August 28, 1963, in Washington, D.C., in front of 250,000 people, is the best example of this.

Every time he repeats his mantra "I have a dream," he follows it up with a few seconds of silence that invite the auditor to do just that, and the impact is all the more pronounced because his mantra connects with the end of the preceding sentence:

"I have a dream . . .

That one day on the red hills of Georgia, the sons of former slaves and the sons of former slave owners will be able to sit down together at the table of brotherhood. I have a dream that one day even the state of Mississippi, a state sweltering with the heat of injustice, sweltering with the heat of oppression, will be transformed into an oasis of freedom and justice."

Never was there greater harmony, one could almost say symphonic harmony, between content, form, and interpretation. But however magnificent Martin Luther King Jr.'s speech, it still follows the rules of "the voices in power"; here we have a preacher addressing the faithful. However beautifully deserving the cause, it must be said his vocal technique comes in very handy. His silences announce a dream that begs to come true.

If the silence is too short or silences are too frequent, the musicality of the discourse is interrupted, because the auditor isn't given enough time to interiorize what has just been said. Rhythm is the heartbeat of silence.

On *The Daily Show*, the American news satire and talk show program aired by Comedy Central, a synthesized voice is often used to imitate Barack Obama, a staccato, monochord voice that drones on more than it talks. It is an attempt to caricaturize the habit the president of the United States has of losing the harmonics in his voice when he speaks. His pauses are too numerous, too repetitive, and they come at intervals that are too regular. It is as if a metronome were speaking, which weakens his emotional impact. His intonation, as indeed his entire discourse, is dolefully binary. A change of rhythm would be so welcome. And yet, he got elected and reelected. It is a fact that when you hear his speech, you're reminded of Abraham Lincoln, or some other legendary figure in American history, not a vulgar synthesized voice. How does he do that? He presents himself not as a revolutionary but as a founder. The way he pronounces his words appeals to the parental instinct; his words themselves, far from inciting upheavals, appeal to his auditors' creativity. But in my view, his greatest stroke of genius has been to palliate his lack of vocal rhythm by adopting the slogan "Yes we can," three powerful monosyllables that echo in the collective unconscious, like a new "I have a dream."

His isn't an isolated case. Nicolas Sarkozy interrupts his speech every four syllables. Generally speaking, there has been an undeniable acceleration in vocal rhythm these past years. Is it consequent to the prevailing vocal habit of "zapping" (hopping from one short clip to another) or of disjointed information delivery? Our ears can no longer abide long sentences. Our impatience is probably the root cause of it. Today, politicians chisel choice hard-hitting words, which they feed to nonstop news channels that repeat these over and over.

The competition is on for airtime. Today, politicians have 10 minutes in which to make their point. Their silences perforce have to be very short. Our leaders are aware of this. Some could be tempted to read into this a form of verbal manipulation, as this piling on of brief silences incites the auditor to take on board the lesson, the message, without ever questioning it. It is a fact that a longer silence would invite auditors to ponder what they really thought of what was said. This can't happen if silences are short, repetitive, and associated with simple words that invite no discussion.

On television as on the radio, silences have two targets, the journalist and the auditor. Nicholas Sarkozy is brilliant in this respect. When a journalist questions him about a current event that bothers him, he doesn't answer immediately. He manages to convey by his silence not that he is looking for his words but that he is irritated and trying to calm down in order to avoid being disagreeable. The silence turns into a form of suspense. These two muted seconds will be remembered as those in which he dominated his emotions before answering in a tone that hovers between hurt and anger. Is this a strategy of silence? For my part, I couldn't say if it is premeditated or spontaneous: Sarkozy's voice is the voice of affect, of the hypersensitivity of a hyperpresident, his silence more a matter of self-control. It is his way of coming across as spontaneous and intimate, yet authoritative. It is a double-edged sword. On one hand, it underlines the solemnity of the occasion. On the other, it attempts to give importance to what is to follow and promotes reflexion. Silence showcases the discourse.

How should one treat interrogatory sentences that call for silence? It is my belief that they mask fake silences and fall into two categories. They're either too eloquent, the strategy here being to leave the sentence unfinished because the conclusion seems obvious, or they're exclusive, marking a desire to end the discussion.

In the same way that symphonies cannot be written without the silences inscribed on sheet music by means of pauses, semibreves, minims, and crotchets, politicians have at their disposal a rich palette of silences. Our leaders are artists of the voice; they play with notes, chords, and rhythms. Their silences are more than simple rhetorical devices; they're weapons for convincing the masses and, sometimes, for provoking action.

Gandhi studied in England. When he returned to his native India, he had perfectly assimilated not just the English language but also the British culture. Facing His Majesty's troops who had the crowd in the sights of their rifles, he could easily have pronounced a speech and thus rallied them to his cause, yet he remained silent. But he was actively silent. He stood upright, dressed in white, and looked up at the sky with no trace of resignation. He was in a world of empathy, of the imaginary, of creation, of things spiritual, a characteristic that leaders must have if they're to govern. The British forces faced this wall of silence, denser than any words could be, and that was a mark of the crowd's determination and its will not just to resist but to survive. This massive vibrational silence was so powerful that it changed everything. The soldiers lowered their rifles. That silence was one of the most inflexible and effective weapons the 20th century has ever produced. Is Gandhi's memorable silence not the ultimate might of the voice?

An Intimate Conviction

Silence is a fertile ground for an essential mental process central to the formulation of any opinion: an intimate conviction.

Article 353 of the French code of criminal procedure expresses this most clearly, when it says that subject to the requirement for justifying the decision, the law does not require each judge or each member of the jury of an Assize court to justify the means whereby they have convinced themselves, nor does it prescribe them the rules whereby evidence is to be considered full and convincing and a sufficient burden of proof. The law asks them to question themselves in reflective silence and to sincerely seek, in all conscience, what impression was made on their reason by the evidence given against the accused and by the defense arguments and ploys. The law has but one question for them, which contains the full measure of their duties: "Is your conviction beyond reasonable doubt?"

From this mixture between factual, attested elements and intuitive, emotional elements is born the intimate conviction of each juror. But because the justice system appeals to a concept that is by nature immaterial and almost irrational, along the centuries, a complex and elaborate ceremonial has been developed and is respected, allowing the intimate conviction to formulate its truth, which is then validated by society.

The ritual of the Assize court borrows from both the liturgy and the theater. The ceremonial of a criminal investigation with a jury, as still practiced today, is highly reminiscent of one of the greatest tragedies of the antiquity, *The Eumenides*, by Aeschylus.

To judge Orestes for the murder of her mother Clytemnestra, Athena, daughter of Zeus, creates a tribunal of men, for it now behooves mortals and choice citizens to pass judgment, once the sole preserve of the gods, who nevertheless attend the debates presided by the goddess Athena. Before this court, on the one side the plaintiff, represented by the Furies, whose fury threatens Orestes, and on the other Apollo, speaking for the defense. Each party states its case. The power of the voice is born in the world of justice.

After the pleadings, the jury is asked to deliberate, but when the votes are counted, the votes for and against the accused are equal. Athena had forewarned the jury that in the event of a tied vote, she would have the casting vote. She pronounces the acquittal of Orestes. One can quite reasonably interpret this judgment as resulting from Athena's deep-seated conviction of Orestes's innocence.

The Assize court has rules, symbols, an etiquette. The trial must adhere to them rigorously. One cannot rule over a man's life without due solemnity.

The oral nature of the debates seems to be inscribed from the very first seconds in the voice of the bailiff announcing the arrival of the bench. The public then rises as a sign of respect, and the presiding judge enters the courtroom, followed by his assessors and the jury.

In the courtroom, the decor is always the same. On one side, the public, and on the other, behind a balustrade and up on a rostrum, the prosecuting attorney. The judge and his assessors dominate the judicial space. It is a black and red composition. The presiding judge, between his two black-robed assessors, wears a red robe. The prosecuting attorney is in black, as is the attorney for the defense, their robe recalling the cassock of yesteryear, with its 33 buttons—one for each year of Christ's life—which had long been their court apparel. And finally, the sash made out of ermine. In the center of the courtroom, witnesses are called to give evidence and to answer the tribunal's questions. The accused is in his box, his attorney for the defense before him. The jurors in their box are silence personified as they listen in silence. No comment, no sound imitation, no interjection reflecting anger or sadness must leave their lips. At best, their body language may eventually give them away and reveal to the lawyers the silent voice of the intimate conviction they're busy evolving.

When the jury is constituted, each juror must swear an oath according to the terms of Article 304 of the French penal code: "You swear and promise to examine with the most scrupulous attention the charges that will be laid against <the defendant>; to betray neither the interests of the defendant, nor the interests of the society that accuses him, nor the interests of the victim; not to communicate with anybody until you [declare your verdict]; not to listen to hatred, malice, fear or affection; to remember that the defendant is presumed to be innocent and that doubt must benefit him; to decide for yourself according to the charges and the means of defence, according to your conscience and intimate conviction, with the impartiality and firmness that befits an honest and free person, and to keep the secret of the deliberations, even after you cease to be a juror."

Behind the courtroom is the deliberation room, which, like the dark wings of a theater, is far from the public eye. Indeed, the jury's deliberations are confidential, subject to the secrecy rule. No one may enter or leave the holy of holies before a verdict has been reached and finally pronounced out loud by the presiding judge before all assembled. In a sacred and absolute silence, the voice delivering justice resonates fully.

The trial has a beginning and an end. It is irreversible. Whatever is said cannot be deleted. This time constraint reinforces the dramatic intensity of the trial, which is subject to rules of conformity: same décor, same actors, same seating.

The dramatization of justice manifests itself in the fact that all the arguments, without exception, must be oral. The reason for this is very simple. Jurors have no access to any written documentation and may only learn the facts of the case through the spoken interventions in court. The power of the voice and of its silences is therefore absolute. This is why it needs to be channeled, ensuring no one takes the floor without warning. If the accused, a lawyer, the attorney general, a juror, or even an assessor wants to be heard, he must first inform the presiding judge, who may or may not authorize it and who can, at any time, suspend the sitting if he feels that emotion is running too high and that the dignity of the trial is at stake. His word can't be challenged, which is why he must be rigorously neutral and assert his authority solely to ensure the proper conduct of the debates. The presiding judge is master of his voice and master of all voices in his court.

The prosecution has the support of a public prosecutor, the attorney general. As far as the accused and his defense attorney are concerned, the attorney general is "the baddy" who, at the end of the trial, will make his closing speech and call for a usually stiff sanction. If the accused has recognized the facts, the attorney general will charge him without mentioning any attenuating circumstances. Through his voice and words, he will try to sway the jurors by toying with their emotions. If the accused claims his innocence, the attorney general will try to convince the jury of his guilt through a more rational plea.

In the same way, the attorney for the defense will try to play to the jury's emotions in his plea if the accused recognizes the facts; otherwise, he will try to demonstrate rationally that the accused can't have committed the acts he has been accused of.

The innocence plea can be just as coherent as the guilty plea. The jurors, subjected to radically different viewpoints, may be destabilized and convinced in turn by the attorney general's argument and by the defense attorney's argument.

During a trial, the power of the voice and its silences are at their peak, and a number of the rules that were relevant for politicians also apply here. Notably, attorneys must know how to convince all the strata of society. Indeed, it bears reminding that the jury is made up of lay members of the public, whose names have been drawn at random; hence, some of them may be entering a courtroom for the first time and may not have the first idea of how the system works.

The extreme tension and tragic atmosphere that overshadow the oral arguments in court can, under the influence of mirror neurons, trigger a downright emotional storm that liberates the urges, fears, and fantasies of both the jury and the public. This cathartic release is a consequence of the impact of each and every orator, whose vocal power comes into full play.

As experienced professionals, the attorney general and the attorney for the defense use their trial skills to maximize the power of the word and of emotional vibrations, which can plunge the jurors into a kind of hypnotic state. Furthermore, jurors have a duty to sort out, from the flow of voices assailing them, factual information from contrasting emotional sensations and to seek the truth in the depths of their heart in order to judge the case "to the best of their knowledge and belief," with "an intimate conviction," alternately known as "a conviction beyond reasonable doubt."

Like an indelible vibrational tattoo, the voice has the leading role in a trial. It imprints itself in people's minds, impacts their judgment and their reasoning. It solicits the passions of both the public and protagonists. The voice is both an offensive and a defensive weapon, its armor made of rhetoric and eloquence, its munitions stock composed of words, silences, rhythm, and the harmonies of its timbre. Language may be the structure upon which thinking is developed, but the voice imposes itself on our thinking. When the assault is launched in court, the rhythm of the voice becomes binary, almost "military." The attorney general, master of the affective vibration of his argument, is a formidable orator. His commanding eloquence has a style that is all his; it has his stamp on it. It is sui generis; no one can copy it or borrow it. It embodies the aptitude to express in a natural manner the emotion of words, the mystery of silences, the minor or major chord that seems familiar before it has even been heard, listened to, decrypted. Whether he adopts a low or a high register, a faint or a booming voice, it is always in harmony with the audience he seeks to persuade. He knows how to play with silences. Not those mind-numbing silences, but a silence that is engaging. Here, in this courtroom, more than anywhere else, vocal charisma is at work in the depths of our emotional universe.

But the mandatory silence imposed on the public also has its importance. All the actors in the trial are sensitive to it. They use it. They feed off it. They look out for the approval of the gallery that may manifest itself in an eloquent silence, nodding heads, subtle shifts of position, or mutterings. Such is the strength of the silence of the voice. Its power undeniably influences jurors and nourishes their intimate conviction in a story that unfolds minute after minute; contrary to tragedies, it is never written. The verdict is always uncertain. It takes shape, gets fleshed out and elaborated as the trial progresses. Its outcome certainly depends on objective evidence, but it can also be the consequence of the timbre used by the orators, the witnesses, the accused, or any person taking the stand. The reporting of the facts may play a less decisive role than the jurors' psyche. To develop a conviction beyond reasonable doubt, the jurors must first become convinced of the sincerity of the arguments. The jurors' perception of the voice of the accused, of his body language, of everything emanating from him is the first phase of their assessment of his sincerity.

If an intimate conviction is so problematic to define, it could be because by its very wording, it sends us back to two almost opposite realities: reason and emotion. On the one hand, it seems conviction must be built on rational and concrete elements. Is the evidence "exhibits," presented during the trial to bring proof of the guilt or innocence of the accused, not physical objects? On the other hand, what is intimate isn't based on any objects; it stems from the heart of our conscience. Here the adjective "intimate" is no less than the emotional secret of the soul.

But how is this intimate conviction arrived at? It is the fruit of both rhetoric and eloquence.

In this oratory art, rhetoric is essential. Rhetoric is all about technique and skill at manipulating words; it is about managing talent in the space-time continuum of the oratory duel during the presentation of arguments; it is both the science and the technique of influencing the mind through argument.

For its part, eloquence is an art unto itself. Much more than an aptitude to speak brilliantly, it is, as I've already pointed out, the aptitude to express in a natural manner the emotion of words, the mystery of silences, the minor or major chord that seems familiar before it has even been heard, listened to, or decrypted.

This conflict between reason and emotion is a theme that is brilliantly exploited in the film *12 Angry Men*, by Sydney Lumet.

A special feature of Lumet's drama is that it focuses exclusively on the in-camera deliberations of a 12-man jury brought together to establish the guilt or innocence of a young man accused of murdering his father. Quite apart from the staging of the jurors' sometimes stormy and even violent discussions, the film gives the impression that its director has set out to film inside the jurors' conscience in order to reveal the tortuous process whereby jurors develop a conviction beyond reasonable doubt. At the start of the debates, 10 out of the 11 jurors are convinced of the guilt of the accused, yet one juror, played by Henry Fonda, manages to introduce the worm of doubt into the mind of each juror, by attacking their reasoning rather than the person, and thus turns the situation around. There is a constant to-ing and fro-ing between highly rational discussions (such as how does a switchblade knife work) and the most intimate revelations (such as the existing conflict between one of the jurors and his own son).

In 1954, in *Notes sur l'affaire Dominici* (*Notes on the Dominici Case*), Jean Giono writes, "I'm not saying that Gaston Dominici isn't guilty. I'm just saying that I haven't heard the proof that he is. . . . The presiding judge, the assessor, the judges, the attorney general, the counsel for the defence . . . all are convinced beyond reasonable doubt of the guilt of the accused. I say that their conviction hasn't convinced me."

Based on the same trial elements, the same proof brought before the court, Jean Giono forged an intimate conviction that was diametrically opposite to the one held by the magistrates, whose honesty, sincerity, and professional probity he did not doubt.

Jean Giono thought that the unfolding of the trial and its outcome hinged on a number of linguistic misunderstandings between the Dominici clan and the rest of the courtroom. The writer observes that Gaston Dominici used a total of 35 words:

"Not one more, I counted them." And he added, "Any other accused man with a vocabulary of two thousand words would have come out of that trial pretty much without blemish. If on top of that, he had had certain eloquence, the gift of the gab, he would have been acquitted. Despite his confession." Giono systematically points out the misunderstandings, the shifts in meaning, and the hasty transcriptions that step by step contributed to the jury's conviction "beyond a reasonable doubt."

The constraint of the ruling that imposes a unanimous verdict, a constraint that forces several voices to become but one, obliges jurors to evaluate the evidence from a single angle, without any nuance. When conviction beyond a reasonable doubt is nothing more than a coalescence of subjectivity between jurors, danger threatens.

The silence at work in the depths of the conscience to arrive at an intimate conviction is somewhat reminiscent of the silent cry of the empty page. When Emile Zola, on January 13, 1898, expressed on the front page of the daily newspaper *L'Aurore* his intimate conviction concerning the innocence of Captain Dreyfus, he used a judicial expression: his "J'accuse" (I accuse), though couched on paper, resonates so strongly that it is a wake-up call for justice. In his open letter to the President Felix Faure, Emile Zola enables the power of his written word to be heard with all its vibrations. He uses all the tricks and skills of the oratory art so well that even today, his writing is listened to rather than read.

He talks in the first person and commits himself unstintingly in the text in which all the verbs are action verbs. His determination comes through in his use of firm, energetic, and precise expressions that come straight to the point. He takes risks. He says so, he knows so. His "J'accuse" (I accuse), hammered home time and time again, does not tolerate any comeback; it is both a plea and an indictment.

Emile Zola engages his readers and exhorts them to take a stand. His style is declamatory and not without irony, a weapon Zola had purposefully chosen to serve his written jousting in which his oral stamp is omnipresent. The rhythm of his text is the rhythm of spoken language. One can almost hear him catching his breath. "J'accuse" is an exceptional example of oratory eloquence, and yet it is a written text. Better than had it been recorded, Zola's voice has withstood the test of time for over a hundred years now.

The Verdict of the Clock

Two o'clock in the afternoon. Marseille is bathed in blazing sunshine when the trial opens on this June day. The courtroom is full, the atmosphere electric. Despite the whirring ceiling fans, it is very hot in the courthouse. The accused is already in place, alone in his box. Badly shaven, his head between his hands, face somber and disheveled, he is wearing a gray jacket, black trousers, and a blue shirt. In the general hubbub in which people are commenting freely, the trial begins. The bailiff escorts the presiding judge and the two magistrates in and announces out loud, "The court!" Everyone rises. A solemn silence reigns. The protocol is impressive. The president in his red dress and his two assessors in their black robes take place on the bench that forms a veritable raised rampart, from which they dominate the courtroom and whence the verdict shall fall. The prosecuting attorney and the counsel for the defense, also in black robes, take their place next. The nine jurors—artisans, teachers, or traders—drawn by lot, are seated in the jury box. These simple citizens must shoulder the responsibility for judging this man, slumped on his bench.

The trial begins. All proceedings are oral. The voice has the power to convict an innocent man or to exonerate a guilty person. Its vibrations are the weapon in this battle. The power of this voice depends on finding a middle road between chaos and harmony, coherence and stupefaction, rupture and compromise. The president asks the accused to stand and state his name, profession, date of birth, and his residence at the time of the deeds he is being charged with. The moment is intense. The jurors are going to get acquainted with the accused through his voice, which will reveal to the court and to the public his affective universe. Should his voice be unpleasant, he will be presumed guilty; should it be pleasant, he will be presumed innocent. The name of the accused has just rung out; he perks up. He now exists.

Another voice is now heard. The courtroom clerk reads the indictment prepared by the prosecutor on the basis of the facts established by the investigating detectives of the Marseilles police force, the forensic experts, and the testimony of certain witnesses.

"Towards 6 p.m., at their home, in their kitchen, Mr. Paul Dupond, aged 36, grabs a knife and stabs his wife four times, thrice in the abdomen, once in the lungs. Then he takes a plastic bag and places it over the head of Mrs. Dupond, aged 32. He tightens the bag around her neck with a thong in order not to hear the moans of his agonizing wife, till death ensued."

Witness after witness testifies on the witness stand. Their voice, attitudes, or looks will confirm the affirmations of the prosecution or of the defense counsel. If need be, a few photos may illustrate the debate.

Not a single line may be read. In this context, only vocal pulses, intonations, and silences may prevail. Between testimonies, the prosecutor pursues his precise and aggressive interrogation. His orator's voice resonates in the courtroom.

In 1912, André Gide wrote in his book *Souvenirs de la cour d'assises* (*Memories of the Assize Court*), "The jurors are glued to their seat by the power of the oral pleas." The prosecuting attorney now rises. Imposing, solemn, his voice becomes an arc, his words like arrows wounding, cutting, and potentially fatal. The president, the defense attorney, the prosecutor, the accused, and the public listen to him in complete silence. His voice, conveyor of morals and emotions, is his weapon. One he knows how to use. When the word is authoritarian, it perforce accuses. It is a strategy. If the plea is too long, the voice tires and loses its impact; if the voice is badly placed, the plea is less effective, and the power of persuasion dwindles. He therefore maintains a particular vocal timbre that is twixt harmony and strife, between a break in rhythm and perfect rhythm. He concludes with force, vigor, and conviction. In an impressive silence that he has appropriated, he advocates the sanction he deems appropriate.

The defense attorney now rises. The oratory jousting can now begin. Each word counts.

The president, his two assessors, and the prosecuting attorney dominate the courtroom. It is a duel and the verb has taken the place of the sword. The indictment was so shocking that everyone is impatient to hear the defense attorney's first words or, rather, the first harmonics of his voice. Will he be convincing? But it's not yet time for his defense plea. He must first hook his audience. Paradoxically, it's the silence that follows the first words that reveals if the timbre is right, if the power is present, neither too strong nor too weak. If too strong, it is detrimental to understanding the message and makes listening painful. If too weak, the auditor isn't captivated, and he becomes lost in his own thoughts. A plea is just that, words, rhythm, and silence. Emotion plays as important a role as do the arguments. A bond must be forged with the jury, their language must be spoken, their looks understood.

After an argument in which rhetoric and eloquence have dominated, the defense attorney comes to the conclusion that the wife of the accused was cheating on him, indicating to the jury a potential new line of defense, the crime of passion. The accused has the last word; he answers with surprising self-confidence, and yet. . . .

When the jury retires to deliberate while the public awaits a verdict outside, everyone is well aware of the damning report of the forensic expert. His medical report sounded like a death knell in the courtroom: "Following the autopsy of Mrs. Dupond Colette, aged 32, we found that her death did not ensue from the stabbing, specifically the four stab wounds, but from choking to death over a period of one minute and five seconds." The prosecuting attorney then has a 1-meter-high clock brought in to the courtroom. "Ladies and gentlemen of the jury, members of the public, we will now listen to this clock for sixty-five seconds." The pendulum begins to oscillate. In the courtroom, the silence is heavy and soon becomes harrowing. The silence talks through this regular tic-tac. The last 10 seconds are unbearable. The prosecutor just has to sum up: "You have just lived through the agony of this poor woman." The verdict falls: guilty, with no attenuating circumstances.

Is the power of silence not the ultimate power of the voice?

CONCLUSION

The Future in Search of a Voice

Our exploration of the power of the voice ended with a moment of silence favorable to introspection and to finding our inner voice, otherwise known as our secret garden. Yet neurophysiology is on the brink of violating this secret garden. Indeed, the technique called electrocorticography allows one to record the activity of the brain thanks to electrodes implanted deep below the cranium. We now know that when a person speaks, it automatically activates acoustic waves that harness a network of cells and special neurons located in the inner ear. Voices engaged in conversation can today be deciphered thanks to intracerebral signals that sensors transcribe into graphs. Since voiced sounds and the silent voice both mobilize practically the same neuronal circuits, would it not be possible to decipher that inner voice, using these same sensors? If that were the case, one could then "hear" someone who can no longer talk or who refuses to talk because of a trauma, as occurs in psychogenic aphonia or locked-in syndrome. Very promising research is being done in this field by Professor Brian Pasley at Berkeley, as well as by Stephanie Martin and her team in Lausanne. Perhaps one day soon, an audio helmet will allow one to hear the inner voice, the silent voice. These technological advances pose the question of the nature of the power of the voice in the future.

The concept of vocal recognition is as old as computer technology. For the past 40 years, we've been seeking to control objects through vocal commands. This revolution has been announced several times but has never been properly exploited, despite the fact that the human voice is the most natural interface there can be between us humans and technology. Today, we're limited to sending short vocal messages, but in the future, vocal recognition will be able to command connected objects (a watch, a car, a thermostat, a refrigerator). The voice is even experiencing a big comeback with instant messaging. A simple vocal message, 10 to 15 seconds long, can convey an idea, a tone, an emotion more effectively, more naturally, and faster than the keyboard.

In our complex technological environment, the voice seems to be the simplest means at our disposal to influence our daily life. The revolution of voice-activated personal assistance is under way thanks to smartphone applications. One can identify a song just by humming it into the phone, even if it is hummed offkey! No parameter escapes this super-ear. Our hearing guides our voice and we can shut our eyes to avoid seeing, but our eardrums have no eyelids, though they do filter our hearing.

Until now, voice-activated assistants first identified the words spoken, then analyzed their meaning. The trend now is to combine these two steps.

Talking to an inanimate object that doesn't answer you or else answers in a somewhat unnatural voice can seem bizarre, and generally speaking, talking to a machine doesn't come naturally. But habits change; synthetic voices are improving, sounding more "natural," and the technology for interacting with virtual assistants, that is, with objects connected to the Internet with no screen or keyboard, has been almost fully developed.

Besides improving our creature comforts in the home and impacting our daily life, the power of the voice in the future has since long been studied by Ircam, a French institute dedicated to the research and creation of contemporary music. Ircam is able to not only transform a sung sound but also to synthesize a voice. The objective of speech synthesis is to produce a voice that is as close as possible to the original human voice. What is at stake here is the notion of vocal identity, in other words, the vocal signature of the individual.

In this context and in the interest of an experiment, André Dussolier gracefully agreed to be dispossessed of his gorgeous voice! Several hours of recording were necessary before his voice could be fully synthesized. These recordings were split up into words, syllables, and phonemes, and their characteristics were then analyzed and gathered with the objective of assembling a databank from which any word, as well as a variety of pronunciations, could be generated with the most natural rendering possible. A person's vocal signature is his or her prosody, an intellectual system that naturally associates not only phonemes but also rhythms, pauses, and intonations. The challenge posed by this technology was to model André Dussolier's way of speaking. By tweaking the timbre, one can fashion the expression and emotion of the vocal output. Thus, one can hear a synthesized Dussolier telling the story of Little Red Riding Hood. Amazed, the comedian admitted that even his close family wouldn't be able to tell the difference between his own voice and his synthesized voice.

The genius Stephen Hawking, who for many years hasn't been able to produce any sounds because of his illness, uses a vocal synthesizer. Though he could benefit today from more advanced technology that would give a more natural rendering of his voice, it seems he prefers to carry on with this "cyborg" voice that has become his true vocal identity. Frankly, I'm not entirely surprised, and this extreme example underlines the complexity, ambivalence, uniqueness, and subtlety of our relationship with what gives us our vocal identity.

Nowadays, one person's voice can even be transformed into someone else's; this involves applying a sort of numerical mask that uses the same principles as speech synthesis, only much faster and better, resulting in astounding imitations. This technology was used, for example, to reconstitute the voice of Marshal Pétain for Philippe Saada's film *Juger Pétain*. Mute images as well as transcripts from Pétain's trial were available. All it took to realize Pétain's voice was the application of this numeric mask to an anonymous voice. Similarly, for an exhibition by the artist Philip Parreno, Ircam managed to create a perfect illusion of Marilyn Monroe reading out loud her intimate diary, which of course she had never recorded.

We are indeed on a slippery slope. If our voice is a key element of our identity, it cannot be placed in anyone's hands. The identity of the voice cannot be dissociated from ethical concerns.

In the same way, we can't really talk of the vocal imprint in the same way as we talk of a fingerprint. In criminal cases, the voice may be called on as evidence, using the services of voice experts whose task is to validate the recordings produced in evidence. This despite the fact that the technology for voice recognition doesn't always allow a voice to be formally attributed. In serious criminal cases, this poses a major problem. There are limits that shouldn't be transgressed.

Vocal manipulation has unleashed every fantasy, inspiring forays into science fiction and its temptations. Stanley Kubrik's film *2001: A Space Odyssey* already explored the deviances that artificial intelligence might engender. *Her*, the film by Spike Jonze, portrays an intimate relationship between a human and a computer program. It is a modern variation on Jean Cocteau's play, *La voix humaine*. But whereas in the play, turned into a film by Roberto Rossellini, the object of the central character's love is never seen nor heard by the audience, in *Her*, one can hear the voice of the entity that the male central character is in love with (a sophisticated female voice that has the additional charm of belonging to Scarlett Johansson). In the near future described in the film, the character played by Joaquin Phoenix works for a website and his job is to write love letters on behalf of others in a world in which feelings and writing are dying out. Depressed by his pending divorce, he invests in an intelligent talking operating system to keep him company. He bonds with this female voice that he talks to over the phone and falls in love. The viewer would like to believe in this love story, even if its demise is expected or at least programmed. But one day, he discovers that the sole focus of his fantasy is also the vocal companion of thousands of other phone correspondents. A beautiful love story ends. Will we some day suffer when we lose the voice of our robot? In the future, will we have to recognize that artificial voices have an existence of their own? Will reality go beyond fiction?

After the experiment that left my friend André Dussolier without a voice, he dared to face the question of creation: "There is still something of Man left, albeit a very small part," he conceded with a smile.

Indeed, even if a superhuman voice challenges us to reexamine art and our human limits, I'd like to believe that it could never be compared to the voice of a live being struggling to produce the correct note and perfect intonation.

Since the first pages of this book, I have insisted on the emotional health of the voice. Emotion is a universal language, beyond meaning; this vibration that the voice conveys is what remains and is shared. We will always recall hearing Martin Luther King Jr.'s emotional music, so unique and irreplaceable, and his message of love and peace. Would one have to be deaf in order to want to kill him?

La Callas and the Aborigine's Story

Are you familiar with the documentary in which journalists showed Aborigines some films and video in which Western civilization had been condensed to show it at its best and at its worst, inviting them to comment on it? Thus they viewed image after image: the first men on the moon, French gardens, war scenes, snow, and so on. Generally speaking, they seemed indifferent to our specificities. Until that one day!

The distribution of a very special musical video: The Aborigines looked at The Beatles, Ray Charles, and Michael Jackson and had no strong reaction, just a smile, a nodding. But when the concert by Maria Callas, interpreting "Casta Diva," a sublime aria from *Norma*, Bellini's opera, was shown, they did not understand a word, but they all cried with emotion. The voice of Maria Callas, the *nec plus ultra* of civilized sound, found an echo in these almost naked men with painted bodies, gathered in their huts. The voice is beyond culture dependent, and this is what the Aborigines had to say: "This music isn't of our culture, we don't know what it means, we can only look and listen, but it moves us." And also: "I find it very poignant, though I can't understand it, you get the sense of something sacred." The sanctity of the voice is what makes us human and gives us the potential to surpass ourselves. If the power of the voice exists, it is in those uncertain and magical spheres that we must look for it.